Register N
Access to Your Book!

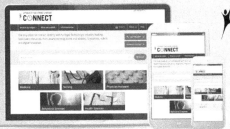

SPRINGER PUBLISHING COMPANY
CƆNNECT™

Your print purchase of *The Physician Assistant Student's Guide to the Clinical Year: Behavioral Health* **includes online access to the contents of your book**—increasing accessibility, portability, and searchability!

Access today at:

http://connect.springerpub.com/content/book/978-0-8261-9538-8
or scan the QR code at the right with your smartphone
and enter the access code below.

AKBNF50V

*Scan here for
quick access.*

If you are experiencing problems accessing the digital component of this product, please contact our customer service department at cs@springerpub.com

The online access with your print purchase is available at the publisher's discretion and may be removed at any time without notice.

Publisher's Note: New and used products purchased from third-party sellers are not guaranteed for quality, authenticity, or access to any included digital components.

THE PHYSICIAN ASSISTANT STUDENT'S GUIDE

to the Clinical Year

BEHAVIORAL HEALTH

Jill Cavalet, DHSc, PA-C, is an associate clinical professor in the Physician Assistant Department at Saint Francis University in Pennsylvania. Dr. Cavalet received a bachelor of science degree in physician assistant science from Saint Francis College. She was a full-time clinical practitioner in the Behavioral Medicine Department at Altoona Hospital and also served as a preceptor. Upon her faculty appointment, Dr. Cavalet received a master of health science degree from Saint Francis University and later a doctor of health science degree from Nova Southeastern University. She continues to precept and practice clinically in behavioral medicine at UPMC Altoona Hospital.

Dr. Cavalet has presented at the state and national levels and has authored many publications. She is a past recipient of the Preceptor of the Year Award from the Saint Francis University Physician Assistant Department and was a finalist in the Saint Francis University Distinguished Faculty Award. She has also been inducted into the Pi Alpha National Physician Assistant Honor Society. Dr. Cavalet has served as a conference proposal reviewer for the American Academy of Physician Assistants, as a subject matter expert for the National Commission on the Certification of Physician Assistants, and as an item writer for the Physician Assistant Education Association.

Maureen Knechtel, MPAS, PA-C (Series Editor), received a bachelor's degree in health science and a master's degree in physician assistant (PA) studies from Duquesne University in Pittsburgh, Pennsylvania. She is the author of the textbook *EKGs for the Nurse Practitioner and Physician Assistant,* first and second editions. Ms. Knechtel is a fellow member of the Physician Assistant Education Association, the American Academy of Physician Assistants, and the Tennessee Academy of Physician Assistants. She is the academic coordinator and an assistant professor with the Milligan College Physician Assistant Program in Johnson City, Tennessee, and practices as a cardiology PA with the Ballad Health Cardiovascular Associates Heart Institute. Ms. Knechtel has been a guest lecturer nationally and locally on topics including EKG interpretation, chronic angina, ischemic and hemorrhagic stroke, hypertension, and mixed hyperlipidemia.

THE PHYSICIAN ASSISTANT STUDENT'S GUIDE

to the Clinical Year

Jill Cavalet, DHSc, PA-C

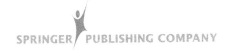

SPRINGER PUBLISHING COMPANY

Springer Publishing Company, LLC
11 West 42nd Street
New York, NY 10036
www.springerpub.com
http://connect.springerpub.com

Acquisitions Editor: Suzanne Toppy
Compositor: diacriTech

ISBN: 978-0-8261-9528-9
ebook ISBN: 978-0-8261-9538-8
DOI: 10.1891/9780826195388

19 20 21 22 / 5 4 3 2 1

The author and the publisher of this Work have made every effort to use sources
believed to be reliable to provide information that is accurate and compatible with the
standards generally accepted at the time of publication. Because medical science is con-
tinually advancing, our knowledge base continues to expand. Therefore, as new information becomes available, changes in procedures become necessary. We recommend that the
reader always consult current research and specific institutional policies before performing any clinical procedure. The author and publisher shall not be liable for any special,
consequential, or exemplary damages resulting, in whole or in part, from the readers' use
of, or reliance on, the information contained in this book. The publisher has no responsibility for the persistence or accuracy of URLs for external or third-party Internet websites
referred to in this publication and does not guarantee that any content on such websites
is, or will remain, accurate or appropriate.

CIP data is on file at the Library of Congress.

Library of Congress Control Number: 2019910958

Contact us to receive discount rates on bulk purchases.
We can also customize our books to meet your needs.
For more information please contact: sales@springerpub.com

Publisher's Note: New and used products purchased from third-party sellers are not
guaranteed for quality, authenticity, or access to any included digital components.

Printed in the United States of America.

To the memory of Cathryn Vargo and to Craig, Madison, and Avery, for your patience and support.

—JILL CAVALET

Contents

e-Chapter 8. Case Studies in Psychiatry
https://connect.springerpub.com/content/book/978-0-8261
-9538-8/chapter/ch08

e-Chapter 9. Psychiatry Review Questions
https://connect.springerpub.com/content/book/978-0-8261
-9538-8/chapter/ch09

Peer Reviewers

Wallace Boeve, EdD, PA-C   Professor and Program Director, Physician Assistant Program, Bethel University, Saint Paul, Minnesota

Rebecca L. McClough, MPAS, PA-C   Director of Clinical Education, Harris Department of Physician Assistant Studies, Wingate University, Wingate, North Carolina

Preface

For a physician assistant student, the clinical year marks a time of great excitement and anticipation. It is a time to hone the skills you have learned in your didactic training and work toward becoming a competent and confident healthcare provider. After many intense semesters in the classroom, you will have the privilege of participating in the practice of medicine. Each rotation will reinforce, refine, and enhance your knowledge and skills through exposure and repetition. When you look back on this time, you will likely relish the opportunities, experiences, and people involved along the way. You may find an affinity for a medical specialty you did not realize you enjoyed. You will meet lifelong professional mentors and friends. You may even be hired for your first job.

Although excitement is the overlying theme, some amount of uncertainty is bound to be present as you progress from rotation to rotation, moving through the various medical specialties. You have gained a vast knowledge base during your didactic training, but you may be unsure of how to utilize it in a fast-paced clinical environment. As a clinical-year physician assistant student, you are not expected to know everything, but you are expected to seek out resources that can complement what you will learn through hands-on experience. Through an organized and predictable approach, this book series serves as a guide and companion to help you feel prepared for what you will encounter during the clinical year.

Each book was written by physician assistant educators, clinicians, and preceptors who are experts in their respective fields. Their knowledge from years of experience is laid out in the pages before you. Each book will answer questions such as "What does my preceptor want me to know?" "What should I be familiar with prior to this rotation?" and "What can I expect to encounter during this rotation?" This is followed by a guided approach to the clinical decision-making process for common presenting complaints, detailed explanations of common disease entities, and specialty-specific patient education.

Chapters are organized in a way that will allow you to quickly access vital information that can help you recognize, diagnose, and treat commonly seen conditions. You can easily review suggested labs and diagnostic imaging for a suspected diagnosis, find a step-by-step guide to frequently performed procedures, and review urgent management of conditions specific to each rotation. Electronic resources are available for each book. These include case studies with explanations to evaluate your clinical reasoning process and review questions to assist in self-evaluation and preparation for your end-of-rotation examinations as well as the Physician Assistant National Certifying Exam.

As a future physician assistant, you have already committed to being a lifelong learner of medicine. It is my hope that this book series will outline expectations, enhance your medical knowledge base, and provide you with the confidence you need to be successful in your clinical year.

MAUREEN KNECHTEL, MPAS, PA-C
Series Editor
The Physician Assistant Student's Guide to the Clinical Year

Introduction

The Approach to the Patient in Psychiatry

OVERVIEW OF THE PSYCHIATRY ROTATION

WHAT TO EXPECT

If you are apprehensive about your psychiatry rotation, you are not alone. It is different from other rotations, and you may not know what to expect. However, it might turn out to be one of the more interesting rotations you complete. Obtaining clinical experience in psychiatry will improve your skills in the emotional aspects of patient care, regardless of your choice of practice. In addition, psychiatric diseases do not exist in a vacuum: You will encounter patients with psychiatric symptoms, suicide attempts, or substance overdoses in the ED; you will manage depression and anxiety, stress, and grief in primary care, including pediatrics and women's health; you will encounter delirium in postoperative settings and in the ICU. Having an understanding of this foundation will serve you well during your training and beyond. As with many things, the more you prepare yourself beforehand, the less nervous you will be. First, let us start with the basics.

Attitude

As with all rotations, you need to maintain a positive attitude and display an interest in learning, even if this specialty is not one of your favorites. Go into the rotation with an open mind, as you never know what you will enjoy until you experience it. In addition, professional behavior is expected. Be respectful toward the patients, and show appreciation toward the staff for contributing to your learning experience.

Setting

Your rotation may occur within an outpatient setting, inpatient setting, or both. Many individuals, both medical professionals and laypersons, are fearful of the concept of an inpatient psychiatric unit. You need not feel this way. Patients who are violent or acting out can be encountered in any medical setting, and they are in the minority of patients you will see overall.

You might also work with psychiatrists who have further training in specialized areas such as child and adolescent psychiatry, geriatric psychiatry, forensic psychiatry, addictions, or consultation/liaison psychiatry.

Patient Populations

The patient population may vary in age, with exposure to children through elderly adults. Some facilities have child and adolescent floors, whereas others have dementia units, and still others might include general adults. If you are caring for a pediatric population, some knowledge of child development will be helpful. In the elderly population, familiarity with common causes of confusion or dementias is necessary. You should take advantage of all learning opportunities so that your rotation is the most well rounded it can be regarding exposure to patient populations.

Responsibilities

Your duties will not differ greatly despite the potential variation in settings or patient populations. The most common duties you will have during this rotation are:

- *History taking*
  As with any other rotation, you should expect to gather a patient history. The components of the psychiatric history are further outlined later in this introduction.

- *Mental status examination (MSE)*
  This is a rotation-specific evaluation that you should be prepared to master. The MSE generally takes the place of the physical

examination in psychiatric settings. The MSE is discussed in detail in the Pertinent Psychiatric Examinations section later in this introduction.

- *Physical examinations*

  Although the MSE is an important objective assessment in psychiatry, the role of the physical examination should not be diminished. In most outpatient psychiatric settings, the evaluation and maintenance of physical health are left to a primary care provider. On an inpatient unit, however, you might be expected to perform physical examinations on new admissions or for problem-specific complaints. This will differ by site. Note that you may also need to adjust your usual head-to-toe examination in certain patients. Those who are anxious, paranoid, or manic, for example, may require you to defer certain components or proceed in a different order than what you are used to.

- *Formulating a diagnosis and treatment plan*

  You should be able to construct a differential list that can be further refined into a final diagnosis. The *Diagnostic and Statistical Manual of Mental Disorders*, Fifth Edition (*DSM-5*), is published by the American Psychiatric Association and is the most appropriate resource for diagnostic criteria.[1] You should familiarize yourself with this text if you have not already.

  Remember that there are no diagnostic tests or procedures to confirm psychiatric diagnoses. Once you become more comfortable with your diagnostic skills, you can then develop treatment plans for patients you have evaluated independently or have seen in conjunction with your preceptor.

- *Presenting to your preceptor*

  Presentations are a standard component of any rotation, and psychiatry is no different. In this setting, you will focus on the pertinent psychiatric history, MSE, substance use history, and family psychiatric history in addition to the past medical history.

- *Managing medical illnesses*

  You may be asked to evaluate medical concerns of patients hospitalized on a psychiatric unit. You could also find yourself taking care of the medical needs of psychiatric patients while on a general internal medicine or hospitalist rotation. This is an excellent way to practice integrating your medical and psychiatric knowledge.

- *Consultations*

  You will potentially have the opportunity to complete psychiatric consultations on a medical inpatient floor. Consults may be ordered for a variety of reasons, including management of psychiatric medications or assessment of suicidal ideation. You may determine that once medically stable, a patient is in need of transfer to the psychiatric unit for further inpatient care. The content and format of a consultation are similar to the admission psychiatric history discussed as follows.

- *Documentation*
  As with other rotations, you may be given access to the medical record for documentation. Be prepared to handwrite notes in case electronic systems are down. Inpatient documentation can consist of progress notes, inpatient admissions or discharge summaries, or consultations. Outpatient documentation will include new-patient evaluations as well as progress notes for follow-up visits.

- *Meetings*
  Your attendance at inpatient treatment team meetings might be expected. A multidisciplinary team approach is common on inpatient psychiatric units, and regular treatment team meetings are held to review the progress and discharge planning of patients. Members of the interprofessional staff are discussed as follows.

  In addition, if an involuntary commitment needs to be extended, a legal commitment hearing will occur. This is discussed in the Commitment Status section later in this introduction.

The Psychiatric History

Next, let us outline the psychiatric history-taking process. The history and MSE are the most important components of the patient evaluation. A psychiatric history differs somewhat from a regular medical history. The main components are as follows:[2]

- *Identifying data*
  Indicate the patient's name, age, gender, and race/ethnicity.

- *Source of information*
  Indicate whether the information is from someone other than the patient and whether the source is reliable.

- *Chief complaint*
  You will still elicit a chief complaint as in other areas of medicine, but instead of "chest pain," "rash," or "cough," be prepared to evaluate "suicidal thoughts," "nervousness," or even "I don't know—they forced me to come here!" The chief complaint can be phrased using the patient's words.

- *History of present illness (HPI)*
  Similar to a medical history, you will obtain the story of what brought the patient to the hospital or office. The usual factors of a medical history will not apply to a psychiatric complaint, however. You will not be able to assess the location, quality, or quantity of psychiatric symptoms as you would for a pain complaint. Rather, have the patient describe how he or she is feeling and assess for impairment in functioning. Ascertain what, if any, issues precipitated this episode. Examples include medication noncompliance; stressors at work or school; legal, medical, or financial concerns; or interpersonal problems.

  Also complete a psychiatric review of systems to screen for and construct a differential diagnosis. Inquire about symptoms such as mood disturbances, anxiety, psychosis, substance use, cognitive impairment, eating disorders, trauma, obsessions, inattention, or hyperactivity.

> **CLINICAL PEARL:** The acronym AMPS (anxiety, mood disorders, psychosis, and substance use) can be utilized in considering common differential diagnoses for the review of systems.

- *Past psychiatric history*
  The past psychiatric history should include previous diagnoses and treatment. Knowing the response or adverse reactions to past treatments is valuable in formulating a current plan. Previous hospitalizations and reasons for admission should also be included. If applicable, detail any past suicidal or self-harm (cutting or burning) behaviors as well as treatment for substance use.

- *Social history*
  The social history may include the following factors, as appropriate to the patient or situation and as can be recalled by the patient:
  - Developmental history
    - Milestones met, any delays, mother's use of drugs or alcohol
  - The environment in which the individual was raised
    - Trauma, abuse, neglect, discipline
  - School performance or educational level
    - Learning disabilities, truancy

- ○ Relationship/marital status
  - ▪ Divorced, never married, children, peer relationships
- ○ Current living arrangement
  - ▪ Alone, with family or others
- ○ Legal issues
  - ▪ Charges, arrests, incarcerations, probation, violent behavior
- ○ Employment history
  - ▪ Pattern of stability, terminations
- ○ Military service
  - ▪ Exposure to trauma, discharge status (honorable, dishonorable)
- ○ Sexual history
  - ▪ History of abuse or assault, any dysfunctions, sexual practices
- ○ Religious affiliation
  - ▪ Views on suicide, source of support, adherence to certain beliefs
- ○ Hobbies
  - ▪ Presence of, or any reduced or given up
- ○ Diet and exercise
  - ▪ Current or past patterns
- ○ Illicit drug use and alcohol
  - ▪ Substances used and in what amount/frequency
- ○ Support system
  - ▪ Isolated or good support system
- *Past medical history*
  You should detail a comprehensive past medical history and medication list in addition to the psychiatric history. Many medical comorbidities and/or treatments can cause psychiatric symptoms, increase risk for psychiatric disorders, or affect the treatment plan. It is imperative to understand that medical causes of psychiatric symptoms need to be evaluated and ruled out before any psychiatric diagnosis is given (Box I.1).

Box I.1 Medical Causes of Psychiatric Symptoms

Addison disease

Brain tumors

Central nervous system infections

Cerebrovascular accident

Cushing syndrome

Dehydration

Diabetes

Electrolyte abnormalities

Hepatic disorders

Hyperthyroidism or hypothyroidism

Hypoglycemia

Hypoxia

Intoxication with substances

Lupus

Lyme disease

Multiple sclerosis

Neurosyphilis

Normal pressure hydrocephalus

Parkinson disease

Pheochromocytoma

Renal disease

Seizures

Toxin exposures

Traumatic brain injuries

Vitamin deficiencies

Withdrawal from substances

Source: From Sadock BJ, Sadock VA, Ruiz P. *Kaplan and Sadock's Synopsis of Psychiatry.* 11th ed. Philadelphia, PA: Wolters Kluwer; 2015.

- *Family history*
  You will want to inquire about a family history of mental illness, hospitalizations, suicide, or substance use. There is a significant genetic and familial risk for many psychiatric disorders. In addition, knowledge about effective medications in family members can assist with pharmacological choices.

> **CLINICAL PEARL:** If a medication has been efficacious for a relative, it may also work well for the patient.[2]

- *Obstacles to history taking*
  Note that you might not be able to gather all of the subjective information that you need or are used to obtaining in other settings.

  ○ Patients with depression might not have the interest or energy to answer questions.

  ○ Patients experiencing mania might not be able to tolerate a lengthy conversation or stay seated.

  ○ Anxious patients might need reassurance and a calming presence during the interview.

  ○ Patients with psychosis can be disorganized in their thinking and speech. They can also be experiencing hallucinations at the time of the interview and appear distracted. Those experiencing paranoia might be outright fearful, or vague and evasive.

  ○ Cognitive impairments also make it difficult to obtain a history. Depending upon the status of the patient, you may have to defer additional history gathering to a later time or use additional sources to corroborate the history.

  ○ Deceptive patients can be seen in any clinical setting; therefore, be aware that patients might lie or falsify information during the evaluation. Motivation might be for secondary gain as in malingering (to obtain medication, avoid legal obligations, etc.) or to assume the sick role as in factitious disorder. Beyond these instances, there might be other reasons that lead patients to being untruthful; thus if there is a question as to the reliability of the source, collateral information should be obtained from others if possible.

Refer to Box I.2 for an outline of the psychiatric history.

Box I.2 The Psychiatric History

Identifying information

Source of data / reliability

Chief complaint

History of present illness

Past psychiatric history, including substance use history

Social history

Past medical history

Family history

Review of systems

WHAT YOUR PRECEPTOR WANTS YOU TO KNOW

In addition to the responsibilities listed earlier, the following are further concepts you will be expected to know:

Commitment Status

- Admissions to psychiatric facilities in the United States involve commitments, either on a voluntary or involuntary basis. Some psychiatric illnesses impair insight, which lead to the need for an involuntary (civil) commitment when the patient refuses to sign himself or herself in on a voluntary basis.[2,3] An involuntary commitment may also be referred to as a psychiatric "hold." The length of time of the commitment varies by state, but one of the common maximum time frames is 72 hours.

- Each state has developed criteria that need to be met for commitment/hospitalization. In most states, the grounds for involuntary commitment involve an imminent threat of potential danger to self or others as a result of a mental illness and/or that the illness impairs the individual to the extent that he or she cannot care for himself or herself.[2,3]

The History of Psychiatric Illness

- Understanding the historical developments regarding mental illness and current perspectives on etiology and treatment may assist you on your rotation. Unfortunately, stigma regarding psychiatric disease still exists today, and the origins of this can be traced back in time. Please refer to Chapter 4, Patient Education and Counseling, for a discussion of psychiatric myths that can be addressed with patients to further assist in destigmatizing psychiatric illnesses.

- In ancient Greece, it was believed that mental illness was caused by the gods. Anyone who was ill or behaving differently received religious treatment. Hippocrates altered this thinking when he postulated that illnesses were due to a disruption in the four humors (body fluids). Throughout the Middle Ages, views on mental illness reverted back to religious themes, and individuals were believed to be possessed or were being punished for immoral behavior. Women with mental illness were victims of witch hunts.[4]

- Continued stigma led to the confinement of individuals in asylums. Previously, patients were hidden or isolated from society either by the law or by their families, who wanted to avoid shame. By the late 1800s, a connection between brain pathology and mental illness was understood, but institutions did little to effectively treat patients, and individuals suffered in deplorable conditions.[4]

- In the early 1900s, Freud's use of psychoanalysis as a form of treatment provided a much different treatment approach. Shock therapy, lobotomies, and other procedures were commonly utilized in the treatment of mental illness until the advent of pharmacotherapy, such as lithium and chlorpromazine administration around 1950. By this time in the United States, exposure of the destitute conditions and inhumane treatments led to the deinstitutionalization of patients and the transfer of care to outpatient settings.[4]

Etiology of Psychiatric Illness

- Psychiatric diseases are thought to be caused by the confluence of a variety of biological, psychological, and social/environmental factors.

- Biological factors include genetics, neurotransmitters, anatomical defects, or brain injury secondary to trauma, toxin exposures, or infections.

- Psychological factors can include trauma, neglect, and early loss of a parent.

- Environmental factors include stressors such as a death, divorce, job loss or change, transfer to a new school, or relationship stressors.[1,2]

Psychopharmacology and Psychotherapy

- It is essential that you are at least familiar with the common pharmacologic treatments in psychiatry. Your knowledge will undoubtedly improve throughout the rotation, but you should have a basic understanding of the most common medications, including their indications.

- Know your drug classes, including antidepressants, mood stabilizers, anxiolytics, antipsychotics, and stimulants. Be able to name specific examples of drugs within the classes and their common side effect profiles. See Chapter 4, Patient Education and Counseling, for further information on pharmacotherapy side effects.

- You should also review common psychotherapy modalities, such as cognitive behavior therapy and dialectical behavior therapy, prior to the rotation. These are discussed further within Chapter 6, Common Procedures and Psychotherapies in Psychiatry.

Medication-Assisted Treatment

- Medication-assisted treatment (MAT) is the use of medications in the treatment of substance use disorders. Amid the current opioid epidemic, MAT commonly refers to the treatment of opioid use disorder; however, MAT can also be used for alcohol use disorder.

- Methadone, buprenorphine, and naltrexone are used in the treatment of opioid use disorder.[2]

- Currently, physician assistants (PAs) can apply for a waiver through the Drug Enforcement Agency (DEA) to prescribe buprenorphine following completion of training by an approved organization.

- Methadone is dispensed through a certified opioid treatment program (OTP).

- Regarding alcohol use disorder, disulfiram, acamprosate, and naltrexone are commonly used medications.[2]

WHAT PREVIOUS PA STUDENTS WISH THEY KNEW BEFORE THIS ROTATION

The Basics

- It is normal to feel overwhelmed or out of place at the start of every rotation. Give it a few days and you will get into the routine. Ideally, you should observe your psychiatric preceptor conducting interviews to obtain a history or accompany the preceptor on rounds before you practice your own skills.

- As with all rotations, know when, where, and with whom you are meeting the first day.

- Prior to arriving, inquire about the dress code and equipment to bring. You should expect professional dress on a psychiatric rotation. You should avoid long or dangling jewelry and scarves. Your white coat might be optional. Avoid clothing that is revealing or is not a proper fit. Wear comfortable but appropriate shoes.

- If you are going to be completing physical exams, you can choose to bring your own equipment or ask whether any is available at the site.

- Be prepared for rounds or patient presentations. Review the chart and become knowledgeable about aspects of the case such as results of diagnostic testing, reports from the previous shift, or new admissions.

Inpatient Unit Guidelines

- One of the first concepts to understand about an inpatient psychiatric unit is that the patients are mobile. Unlike a standard medical floor, you will encounter patients walking around, possibly approaching you, and otherwise being present outside of their rooms.

- Next, be aware of safety procedures. You need to be careful on an inpatient unit, but not fearful. Some patients might display odd or disorganized behaviors due to their underlying illness. These behaviors should not be stigmatized any more than those that patients with medical illnesses experience.

- One of the most common guidelines on an inpatient unit is to place yourself between the patient and the door during interactions. If you are in an office or a patient's room and the patient becomes upset or agitated, you will have a way out. In addition, do not approach patients alone if they have recently been violent or acting out.

- Patients should not have access to potentially harmful items such as sharp objects, belts, or shoelaces. Although there may not be an actively suicidal patient on the unit, these standard safety procedures remain in place at all times. If you are not sure whether you can obtain something for a patient, just ask the staff.

- If you are unsure how to respond to a psychotic patient, a threat, or other uncomfortable situation, be sure to seek help or consultation. Hospital police or other inpatient or outpatient security staff can be called upon as well if needed.

Ask the Staff, and Assist the Staff

- Utilize the knowledge and skill of the staff to answer your questions or concerns. Some of the psychiatrists, nurses, or mental health workers will have many years of experience working with patients with psychiatric illnesses, and they can be one of the best resources available to you.

- In addition, offer to help when you can. Those who enjoy being a preceptor usually know how to utilize a student as an asset and not a burden. Once you are comfortable in the setting, offer to do more not only to assist the staff but to improve your educational experience as well.

How to Respond to Delusions

- A delusion is a false belief. Delusions are not always bizarre and at times sound plausible. A general rule is not to disagree with or challenge a patient who is delusional. That does not mean to agree with the patient either. Instead, ask questions in an attempt to explore the content of the delusion and the effect it is having on the patient.[2]

Be Patient With the Patients

- Those suffering from psychiatric illness may not respond or converse as well as patients on other rotations. Have patience with those who are anxious, depressed, experiencing thought blocking or paranoia, or confused. In addition, provide appropriate empathetic responses to improve rapport with patients.

- Take the time to listen to what the patient is saying. You will likely contribute more to patient care and your own learning experience if you do more listening than talking.

PERTINENT PSYCHIATRIC EXAMINATIONS

Mental Status Examination

The MSE is an objective assessment tool that describes a variety of patient factors at a given time.[1,2] The main components are as follows:

- General appearance and behavior
  - Observe the overall appearance of the patient, including attire, hygiene, eye contact, and facial expressions. Unique findings such as notable tattoos or hair styles may also be included. You can also comment on whether the patient appears to look his or her stated age.
  - Note the patient's behavior/attitude, including degree of cooperation. Observe for any agitation, suspiciousness, hostility, or guarded behavior.
- Motor activity
  - Activity can be slowed, increased, or unremarkable. Observe for restlessness, agitation, or other signs of anxiety, as well as a reduction in activity that may indicate depression. Also note the presence of tremors or unusual postures. Extrapyramidal side effects (EPS) of antipsychotic medications, such as dystonic reactions, akathisia, parkinsonian features, or tardive dyskinesia, might be seen and should be noted as well.
- Speech
  - Note the pace, volume, and fluency of the patient's speech. It might be pressured, as seen in mania, and difficult to interrupt. It might be slow and soft or monotone. Patients who are intoxicated might have slurred speech, whereas other patients may exhibit aphasia or dysarthria.
- Mood and affect
  - Mood is subjective and describes how the patient is feeling. Ask the patient to describe her or his mood or how she or he is feeling.

- Answers might include *happy, sad, depressed, fine, okay, afraid, nervous,* or *irritated,* among others.

○ Affect is objective and is assessed by observing the patient's outward expression.

- Examples include *restricted, blunted,* and *flat,* which indicate varying degrees of a lack of emotional expression.

- A broad affect is used to describe one with a generally normal range of expression.

- A labile affect describes a rapid change in emotion that is unrelated to the environment.

CLINICAL PEARL: A flat affect is a total lack of emotional expression.

○ Also note whether the affect is appropriate (or inappropriate) to the mood and situation. Most of the time the patient's affect will be appropriate to the mood. An inappropriate affect is used to describe a state in which the patient's expression, emotion, or behavior does not align with the situation or content being discussed. For example, a patient who smiles when discussing the recent death of a loved one or a traumatic event would be said to have inappropriate affect. Conditions likely to exhibit inappropriate affect include schizoid personality disorder, dementia, or other organic medical conditions, including those that can cause pseudobulbar affect.

- Perceptual disturbances

○ Perceptual disturbances include illusions and hallucinations.

- Illusions are a misperception of real stimuli.

- You and the patient can both recognize a sensory stimulus, but the patient will perceive it incorrectly. For example, you see a rug on the floor, but the patient misinterprets it as an animal lying still.

- Hallucinations are false sensory perceptions without a real stimulus.

- The patient will sense things that are not there. This can occur in any of the five senses: auditory, visual, tactile, olfactory, or gustatory.

- Hallucinations are much more common than illusions.

○ Perceptual disturbances occur most often in patients with schizophrenia or other psychotic disorders.

○ When evaluating for the presence of either of these perceptual disturbances, you can normalize them because they may be frightening to the patient. The patient may be reluctant to admit to what he or she perceives as an alarming or very abnormal symptom. Inform the patient that, at times, others who are not feeling well and/or are under significant stress may hear sounds or voices that others do not hear, and inquire whether the patient has experienced this as well.

> **CLINICAL PEARL:** Auditory hallucinations are the most common type of hallucination.

○ Command auditory hallucinations are those that tell the patient to do something.[2]

   ▪ A patient who is hearing command auditory hallucinations to harm himself or herself or others should be carefully evaluated for a risk of suicide or homicide.

○ Visual hallucinations are found most often in dementia and delirium.

○ Tactile hallucinations can occur in delirium as well as substance withdrawal.

○ Olfactory hallucinations should prompt an evaluation for a seizure disorder or other medical etiology.

● Thought content

○ Thought content abnormalities include obsessions, compulsions, delusions, ideas of reference, paranoia, phobias, suicidal ideation, and homicidal ideation.

○ Obsessions are intrusive thoughts, urges, or images.

○ Compulsions are repetitive behaviors that an individual performs in response to an obsession.

○ Delusions are fixed beliefs even in the presence of conflicting evidence.

   ▪ Delusions are a symptom of psychosis.

   ▪ Examples of delusional themes include grandiose, persecutory, somatic, and religious.

○ Ideas of reference are when one interprets external events as referring, or having relevance, to them.

○ Paranoia is the belief that one is being persecuted.

○ Phobias are persistent irrational or exaggerated fears.

○ Suicidal ideation is having thoughts about harming or killing oneself or that one would be better off dead.

  ▪ It is extremely important to inquire about this and document whether negative, or follow up if positive. You can start by asking questions such as "Have you thought that life isn't worth living?" or "Have you thought you would be better off dead?" At some point specifically ask whether the patient has *current* thoughts of suicide or of killing himself or herself, and follow up if so.

  ▪ Inquire about a suicide plan and whether patients have taken steps toward furthering it. For example, ask whether they have access to weapons, pills, or other means for potential suicide.

  ▪ If they have experienced past suicidal ideation, inquire as to what has kept them from attempting suicide, and assess for protective factors.

○ Homicidal ideation refers to having thoughts about harming or killing another person. If positive, this needs to be followed up with as well. There is a legal obligation to warn specific individuals if they are threatened.[2] Any previous history of violence should also be gathered. What precipitated or prevented past episodes is also important to explore.

○ Thought insertion is a delusion that outside people or forces are placing thoughts into one's mind. Thought withdrawal is the opposite belief.

○ Thought broadcasting is a delusion that one's thoughts are being broadcasted to the external environment.

• Thought process

  ○ The thought process entails how the patient's thoughts are organized and then expressed in the form of speech or writing.

  ○ A thought process without any abnormalities can be described as linear, coherent, logical, or goal directed.

  ○ Abnormal thought processes include:

    ▪ Circumstantiality

- The speaker includes unnecessary details in speaking or writing and eventually comes back around and gets to the point or answers the question.

- Circumstantial thinking can be seen in patients with schizophrenia or obsessive-compulsive disorder.

CLINICAL PEARL: You can remember this by noting that the prefix *circum* means "around" and that patients with circumstantiality eventually get back around to the point.

- Tangentiality
  - This is similar to circumstantiality, but there is no return to the original point or question; the patient goes off on a tangent.
  - You may need to interrupt and refocus the patient.
  - Tangential thinking can be seen in schizophrenia, bipolar disorder, and other organic brain disorders.

- Loose associations (derailment)
  - Little to no connection is observed between the patient's thoughts. The words form sentences, but the sentences are not connected or goal directed.

- Flight of ideas
  - This refers to rapid shifts of thoughts or ideas, but a logical connection is noted between them.

CLINICAL PEARL: Flight of ideas may be accompanied by pressured speech in patients with mania.

- Perseveration
  - This refers to focusing on an idea or content without being able to move on to other topics. In answering a question, the patient might respond appropriately but then provide the same answer to subsequent questions.
  - Perseveration can occur in dementia, traumatic brain injuries, or schizophrenia.

- Thought blocking
  - This is a disruption in the train of thought or the inability to complete a thought. You may notice the patient stop midsentence. After waiting a short period of time, you can prompt the patient and assist him or her if he or she has forgotten what he or she was saying. In severe thought blocking, it may be difficult to complete the interview.
  - Thought blocking may occur in schizophrenia or depression.
- Neologisms
  - This refers to the creation of new words. The patient may use made-up words or combinations of words that are not real words.
- Word salad
  - This refers to a combination of words that do not form a sentence. The patient who demonstrates significant word salad may be incoherent.
- Clang associations
  - Words are associated by sounds (such as rhyming) and not by meaning.

- Cognition
  Cognition encompasses the mental processes of orientation, memory, language, problem-solving, judgment, and interpersonal relationship and actions.[2] Cognition can be assessed by a formal scored evaluation, such as the Mini-Mental Status Examination, or by a gross evaluation of the following factors:
  - Level of consciousness/alertness
    - This is assessed by observation.
    - Is the patient awake, drowsy, comatose, or other?
  - Orientation
    - Introduce this topic by stating that you will ask several questions to assess memory and thinking.
    - Reassure the patient that this is a common assessment and ask that he or she just tries his or her best.
    - Person: Ask: *What is your full name?*
    - Place: Ask: *Where are we right now?*

- Time: Ask: *What is today's date, including the day of the week?*

- Situation: Ask: *Why are you here?*

> **CLINICAL PEARL:** Make sure to have the patient state the year because this may be the only indicator of disorientation to time if she or he gets the other components correct.

- Concentration
  - Serial 7s (Start at 100 and subtract by 7.)
    - This is intimidating to many patients, but you can encourage them to try. You can stop the patient after approximately five subtractions: (93, 86, 79, 72, 65).
  - You can also attempt subtracting by 3s or counting by 2s to 20.
  - Spell *world* backward.
    - You may need to ensure they can spell it correctly beforehand.
- Memory
  - Tell the patient you are going to check his or her memory.
  - Immediate: Have the patient repeat three words you say to them. The words should be unrelated, such as "ball, cup, dog."
  - Recent: Tell the patient to remember the three words, and ask for the words again in a few minutes. Other options include asking the patient what he or she had for dinner the previous day or who is the current president.
  - Remote: This can be assessed by having the patient state the last several presidents and/or noting whether she or he struggles with remembering past events during the history-taking evaluation.
- As needed
  - Calculation: Have the patient add simple combinations of two-digit numbers or similar examples.

- Fund of knowledge: Assess basic knowledge throughout the interview.
- Abstract reasoning:
  - Assess for the ability to think abstractly as opposed to concretely. Concrete thinking is the inability to grasp another meaning or attain a higher level of analysis.
  - Ask the patient to interpret a proverb, such as "Don't cry over spilled milk." Patients with concrete thinking will have difficulty interpreting the proverb using other words.
  - You can also ask about similarities, such as *How are an apple and an orange the same?* Patients will state simple similarities between an apple and an orange (such as skin or seeds) instead of noting that they are both fruits.

- Insight
  - *Insight* is described as the patient's understanding of his or her illness.
- Judgment
  - Assess whether the patient can problem-solve or make decisions using good judgment. Example questions include *What would you do if you found a stamped, addressed envelope on the sidewalk?* and *What would you do in a movie theater if you smelled smoke?*
- MSE example

A 23-year-old Hispanic female is dressed appropriately and is cooperative. She appears her stated age and makes fair eye contact. She sits still with occasional wringing of hands. Speech is soft but has an appropriate pace. Mood is "sad." Affect is blunted and appropriate to the mood. The patient denies hallucinations and does not appear to be responding to internal stimuli. Thought content is positive for suicidal ideation and negative for homicidal ideation, delusions, obsessions, phobias, or ideas of reference. Thought process is linear without circumstantiality or flight of ideas. Cognition is grossly intact except for minimal difficulty with concentration in serial 7s. Insight is fair, and judgment is impaired. Refer to Box I.3 for an outline of the MSE.

Box I.3 Mental Status Examination Outline

General appearance and behavior

Attire, hygiene, eye contact, facial expressions, appears stated age, level of cooperation

Psychomotor activity

Hyperactive, reduced

Speech

Volume, pace, fluency

Mood

Subjective report

Affect

Objective report; appropriateness to the mood

Thought content

Obsessions, compulsions, delusions, ideas of reference, paranoia, phobias, suicidal ideation, and homicidal ideation

Thought process

Circumstantiality, tangentiality, loose associations, flight of ideas, perseveration, thought blocking, neologisms, word salad, clang associations

Perceptual disturbances

Illusions

Hallucinations: auditory, visual, tactile, olfactory, gustatory

Cognition

Level of consciousness /alertness

Orientation: person, place, time, and situation

Memory: immediate, recent, remote

Concentration

Calculation

Fund of knowledge

Abstract reasoning

Insight

Good, fair, poor

Judgment

Good, fair, poor

INTERPROFESSIONAL STAFF

Mental Health Worker

- This type of staff member can also be referred to as a *psychiatric technician*. He or she engages patients in individual or group therapy, provides assistance with activities of daily living (ADL), and has potentially many other non-nursing duties depending upon the facility.

Nurse

- Nursing staff are an integral component of the psychiatry team as they are in other areas of medicine. You may work with nurses at all levels of training, including psychiatric nurse practitioners.

Occupational Therapist

- Occupational therapists (OTs) might be utilized as part of the multidisciplinary care team. OTs evaluate the patient's ability to perform ADLs, can assess safety concerns, and can lead group therapies.[5]

Psychologist

- You may encounter psychologists during your rotation. Depending upon the level of training, psychologists can provide psychotherapy
and administer and interpret psychological testing (see Chapter 3, Diagnostic Testing). Note that as they are not physicians, they generally cannot prescribe medications, although some states allow limited prescribing authority with additional training.[6]

Recreational Therapist

- Recreational therapists evaluate patients for relaxation and leisure activities. They can also lead groups.[7]

Social Worker

- Social workers or other social services staff assess the patient for discharge planning and coordination of outpatient care. They are integral members of the treatment team. In patients with chronic illnesses, outpatient caseworkers or other staff will be involved in patients' admissions and outpatient care coordination.

CONFIDENTIALITY PRACTICES AND ETHICS

Maintaining confidentiality is as important in psychiatry as in other areas of medicine. When interviewing a patient, a quiet and private area is preferred. In several circumstances, however, confidentiality may be breached: as when child or elder abuse needs to be reported, in some cases of threatened suicide or homicide, if information is court ordered, or for disability evaluations.[2] Note that additional federal confidentiality laws are in place for drug and alcohol treatment programs to encourage patients to seek treatment when they otherwise might be fearful to do so, due to stigma.[2]

Codes of conduct exist to outline expectations for professional and ethical behavior. The four main bioethical principles of autonomy, beneficence, nonmaleficence, and justice need to be considered in the psychiatric setting as well as the medical setting. At times, a patient might be unable to make decisions for himself or herself, and arrangements for guardianship or other conservator provisions need to be made.[2] Recall that competency is a legal determination, but psychiatrists can provide an opinion as to whether a patient has decision-making capacity.

SAMPLE DOCUMENTATION

Admission Note/New Patient Evaluation

The psychiatric admission note (or, if in an outpatient setting, a new psychiatric evaluation) should contain the elements of the psychiatric history outlined earlier. The symptoms that meet criteria for admission (suicidal or homicidal ideation or psychosis/disorganization) should be included if in a hospital setting. In addition, the mental status exam, physical exam, admission labs, and diagnosis are included. Finally, the initial treatment plan should be discussed along with an estimated length of stay or plan for outpatient care.

Discharge Note/Summary

A psychiatric discharge summary differs slightly from a medical discharge note. Include a summary of the patient's hospital stay, with behavior and response to treatment noted. In addition, an updated MSE at the time of discharge, final diagnosis, outpatient appointments, and any follow-up labs need to be included.

Consultation Note

A consultation note is similar to an admission note but also includes the patient's disposition. Indicate whether the patient requires transfer to the inpatient psychiatric unit or can be safely discharged to the outpatient setting once medically stable.

In summary, there is a lot of information to review prior to your psychiatric rotation. You should still have a thorough knowledge base regardless of the rotation setting or your responsibilities. Once in clinical practice, you will likely encounter mental health issues with patients even if psychiatry is not your chosen specialty. Understanding the elements of the psychiatric history and MSE, diagnostic evaluation, and treatment options are key skills in the development of your clinical knowledge.

REFERENCES

1. American Psychiatric Association. *Diagnostic and Statistical Manual of Mental Disorders.* 5th ed. Arlington, VA: American Psychiatric Publishing: Author; 2013.
2. Sadock BJ, Sadock VA, Ruiz P. *Kaplan and Sadock's Synopsis of Psychiatry.* 11th ed. Philadelphia, PA: Wolters Kluwer; 2015.
3. Testa M, West SG. Civil commitment in the United States. *Psychiatry.* 2010;7(10):30–40. https://www.ncbi.nlm.nih.gov/pmc/articles/PMC3392176
4. Farreras IG. History of mental illness. In: Biswas-Diener R, Diener E, eds. *Noba Textbook Series: Psychology.* Champaign, IL: DEF Publishers; 2018. https://nobaproject.com/modules/history-of-mental-illness
5. American Occupational Therapy Association. Occupational therapy's role in community mental health. https://www.aota.org/About-Occupational-Therapy/Professionals/MH/Community-Mental-Health.aspx.
6. American Psychological Association. What do practicing psychologists do? http://www.apa.org/helpcenter/about-psychologists.aspx. Updated July 2014.
7. American Therapeutic Recreation Association. About recreational therapy. https://www.atra-online.com/page/AboutRecTherapy

1

Common Presentations in Psychiatry

Introduction

The psychiatric rotation will provide you with experience that is applicable to any clinical setting. Mastering the ability to listen to the stories that patients will share with you, and to synthesize the information with your observations to formulate a proper diagnosis and treatment plan is an essential skill. The history and mental status examination (MSE) are the keystone of the patient evaluation process in psychiatry.

When presented with a psychiatric chief complaint, there are several steps to follow in order to arrive at the most likely diagnosis:

1. Identify the chief complaint and pertinent past history.

   • Onset, chronology, stressors

   • Pertinent past psychiatric and medical history, surgical history, social history, family psychiatric history, medication and allergy list, and a psychiatric review of systems

2. Create a problem list.

   • Rank problems and identify whether and how they relate to the chief complaint, and separate those problems that do not relate to the chief complaint

3. Summarize pertinent positive and negative findings, both subjective and objective.

   • Perform a thorough history and MSE

4. Formulate and prioritize an appropriate differential diagnosis.

- It is helpful to list the differential diagnoses in descending order of most likely diagnosis; if this step is performed correctly, it should guide the initial management plan; be sure to include "danger differentials," or those that carry a higher mortality risk

5. Initiate a management plan to include diagnostic evaluation and initial treatment, if indicated.

- Order diagnostic studies to establish any medical causes of psychiatric symptoms, establish baseline levels, or to monitor therapeutic drug levels or other pharmacological laboratory monitoring

- Initiate a care plan based on the most likely diagnosis

COMMON PRESENTATIONS

Several common presentations you can expect to encounter in psychiatry include:

Anxiety

Depression

Personality disorders

Psychosis

Substance use disorders

ANXIETY

Anxiety disorders are the most prevalent psychiatric illnesses.[1,2] You will undoubtedly encounter an anxiety presentation during your clinical training in psychiatry and other general rotations. The anxiety disorders can be comorbid with each other and with other psychiatric illnesses, including depression and substance use. Anxiety can be a normal occurrence for many individuals and serves as a warning for a potentially dangerous situation. However, when anxiety becomes pathological and interferes with functioning, it must be evaluated, diagnosed, and treated properly.

Differential Diagnosis

- Adjustment disorder with anxiety
- Generalized anxiety disorder (GAD)
- Obsessive-compulsive disorder (OCD)
- Posttraumatic stress disorder (PTSD)
- Panic disorder
- Selective mutism
- Separation anxiety disorder
- Social anxiety disorder (social phobia)
- Specific phobia
- Anxiety disorder due to another medical condition[1,2]
  - Endocrine
    - Hyperthyroidism, pheochromocytoma, hypoglycemia, Addison disease, Cushing syndrome, others
  - Cardiac
    - Arrhythmias, cardiomyopathy, anemia, others
  - Inflammatory disorders
    - Lupus erythematosus, rheumatoid arthritis, others
  - Neurological
    - Traumatic brain injury, neoplasms, migraine, epilepsy, multiple sclerosis, others
  - Respiratory
    - Chronic obstructive pulmonary disease (COPD), asthma, other hypoxic states
- Substance- or medication-induced anxiety disorder
  - Alcohol withdrawal, caffeine and other amphetamine intoxication, sympathomimetics, others[1,2]

History

- Patients may present with anxiety, fear, worry, or nervousness that has interfered with functioning. The onset and chronology will vary by diagnosis (see Table 1.1).

- The anxiety might be generalized, or occur in specific settings or in response to certain stimuli.

- Patients will most likely experience physical or physiological symptoms of anxiety, including dizziness or lightheadedness, palpitations, diaphoresis, tremors, an upset stomach, or paresthesias. Muscle tension and headache can occur as well.[1,2]

- There may be a history of trauma or another stressor.

- Evaluate for the presence of obsessions and compulsions or panic attacks.

- A medical history and review of medications and/or other substances should be conducted to rule out additional causes of anxiety.

- Inquiring about a past history of anxiety and treatment is important as well.[1,2]

TABLE 1.1 Psychiatric History Specific to Complaint

History	Potential Diagnosis
A significant stressor with distress that exceeds normal expectations	Adjustment disorder with anxiety
Anxiety about a variety of areas with irritability, poor sleep, and muscle tension	Generalized anxiety disorder
Presence of obsessions and compulsions	OCD
Discrete episodes of terror and doom with physical symptoms of anxiety	Panic attack/disorder
A traumatic event followed by intrusive symptoms, avoidance of reminders of the trauma, anxiety, and negative mood state	PTSD
Failure to speak in certain situations	Selective mutism
Fear of separation from a loved one	Separation anxiety disorder
A fear of social situations due to embarrassment	Social anxiety disorder
A specific fear of an object or situation	Specific phobia
Presence of a medication, substance, or medical condition contributing to anxiety	Substance- or medication-induced anxiety disorder

OCD, obsessive-compulsive disorder; PTSD, posttraumatic stress disorder.

Mental Status Examination

The general appearance for a patient presenting with anxiety could include wringing of the hands or fidgeting. The speech might be unremarkable. The mood might be described as worried, nervous, or anxious. The affect should be appropriate to the anxious mood. You should evaluate thought content for obsessions, preoccupations, or phobias. Psychotic symptoms should not be present. The thought process will likely be linear/logical. Concentration may be impaired and insight will vary.[2]

Diagnostic Plan

- You can consider utilizing a clinician- or self-rating scale to help support your suspected diagnosis. The Hamilton Anxiety Rating Scale (HAM-A), Panic Disorder Severity Scale (PDSS), or Yale-Brown Obsessive-Compulsive Scale (Y-BOCS) can be used.[2]
- Order the appropriate diagnostic tests or toxicology screens to evaluate for medical, or medication- or substance-induced causes of anxiety.[2]
  - Complete blood count
  - Comprehensive metabolic panel
  - Thyroid function
  - Brain imaging
  - Others as applicable to rule out specific medical or substance comorbidities

Initial Management

- Overall
  - Evaluate risks for suicide and/or homicide, which may be present in the context of anxiety.
  - Evaluate need for hospitalization versus outpatient treatment.
  - Ensure proper diagnosis and treat accordingly.
  - Psychotherapy and pharmacotherapy alone or in combination are effective for anxiety disorders.[2] This decision can be based upon the severity of the anxiety and patient preference, among others.

- GAD
  - Selective serotonin reuptake inhibitors (SSRIs), buspirone, and venlafaxine (a serotonin–norepinephrine reuptake inhibitor [SNRI]) are recommended. Short-term use of benzodiazepines may be appropriate until the SSRI or the SNRI become fully efficacious.[2,3]
  - Cognitive therapy is recommended, as is behavioral therapy, which includes relaxation techniques and biofeedback.[2,4]
- Panic disorder
  - All SSRIs are efficacious for panic disorder and are recommended as first-line pharmacological treatment. Specifically, paroxetine is U.S. Food and Drug Administration (FDA) approved for panic disorder.[5]
  - Benzodiazepines work more rapidly than other medications but are best used as needed due to concerns with abuse and cognitive impairment. Benzodiazepines can also be utilized short term in bridging therapy while waiting for SSRIs or venlafaxine to become effective.
  - Regarding psychotherapy, there is no evidence that one form is superior over another, but much research has focused on cognitive behavioral therapy.[6]
- Social phobia
  - Cognitive behavioral psychotherapies are effective for social phobia, and can be used alone or in addition to pharmacotherapy.[2,7]
  - Efficacious medications include SSRIs, venlafaxine, or buspirone.[2,8] Benzodiazepines or beta-adrenergic receptor antagonists can be used as needed in exposure situations as well.[2]
- Specific phobia
  - The most commonly used behavior therapy is exposure therapy, specifically, systematic desensitization.[2,9]
  - Pharmacotherapy options include as-needed use of benzodiazepines or beta-adrenergic receptor antagonists.[2] The use of SSRIs or SNRIs would be appropriate if another anxiety disorder is comorbid with specific phobia.
- Other nonpharmacological recommendations for anxiety include obtaining proper sleep, stress reduction, exercise, and reduction/elimination of stimulating drugs, if relevant to the patient.

DEPRESSION

Depression is a common presentation not only in psychiatry but in primary care as well. It can be a symptom of several disorders, and can be accompanied by potentially life-threatening suicidal ideation. Depression needs to be differentiated from normal emotions of sadness or grief.[1,2] A chief complaint of depression requires a careful and thoughtful evaluation to ensure proper diagnosis and treatment.

Differential Diagnosis

- Adjustment disorder with depressed mood
- Major depressive episode/disorder
- Bipolar disorder I or II
- Cyclothymic disorder
- Persistent depressive disorder (dysthymia)
- Adjustment disorder with depressed mood
- Mood disorder due to another medical condition
  - Hypothyroidism, stroke, multiple sclerosis, autoimmune illnesses, Parkinson's disease, epilepsy, others
- Substance- or medication-induced mood disorder
  - Alcohol or central nervous system (CNS) depressants, stimulant withdrawal, antihypertensive drugs
- Somatic symptom disorder
- Neurocognitive disorders (dementia)
- Schizophrenia
- Schizoaffective disorder[1,2]

History

- Patients may present with a chief complaint of depression, or may describe feeling sad, down, or not themselves. The onset and chronology will vary by diagnosis (Table 1.2).
- Anhedonia, or loss of interest or pleasure in activities previously enjoyed, is a common finding as well.

TABLE **1.2** Psychiatric History Specific to Complaint

History	Potential Diagnosis
SIG E CAPS symptoms	Major depressive episode/disorder
Manic symptoms	Bipolar I disorder
Hypomanic symptoms	Bipolar II disorder
Always been depressed	Persistent depressive disorder (dysthymia)
Significant stressor	Adjustment disorder with depressed mood
Mood symptoms prior to onset of menses	Premenstrual dysphoric disorder
Memory or language impairment	Alzheimer disease /dementia
Multiple somatic symptoms with unexplained workup	Somatic symptom disorder
Psychotic symptoms (hallucinations, delusions, or disorganized behavior)	Depression with psychotic features, schizophrenia, or schizoaffective disorder
Substance, medication, or another medical condition	Substance- or medication-induced mood disorder

- Additional symptoms can include sleep and appetite disruption, difficulty concentrating, feelings of guilt, decreased energy, or suicidal ideation.[1,2]

CLINICAL PEARL: The common mnemonic SIG E CAPS can be used to remember the symptoms of a major depressive disorder.

SIG E CAPS
Suicidal thoughts
Interest (loss of); anhedonia
Guilt
Energy (decreased)
Concentration (impaired)
Appetite change
Psychomotor agitation or retardation
Sleep change

- Somatic presentations of depression are more common in the geriatric population.

- Children or adolescents may present with school concerns, irritability, or risky behaviors.

- The history may also contain one or more stressors that precipitated the episode. Anxiety can frequently co-occur with depression as well.[1,2]

- Inquiring about a past history of depression and prior treatment is important as well

> **CLINICAL PEARL:** A first episode of depression might be a manifestation of bipolar disorder. This is more likely in those with a positive family history of bipolar disorder, those with psychotic features, or those with onset in adolescence.[1,2] History taking should inquire about these factors.

Mental Status Examination

The general appearance of a patient presenting with depression might be appropriate, or he or she could display some degree of being disheveled if the patient has not had energy or desire to care for activities of daily living (ADL). He or she may display poor eye contact. The patient will typically be cooperative, but may display a negative outlook or have psychomotor retardation. The speech could be slow and/or soft. Thought content might include suicidal ideation. Psychotic symptoms such as delusions or hallucinations are not typical of depression, but can occur in severe cases. The thought process will likely be linear/logical but can be slowed or exhibit thought blocking. Concentration may be impaired due to lack of energy or interest, and insight will vary.[2]

Diagnostic Plan

- You can consider utilizing a clinician- or self-rating scale to help support your suspected diagnosis. The Hamilton Rating Scale for Depression (HAM-D), Beck Depression Inventory, or Zung Self-Rating Scale are commonly used.[2]

- Order the appropriate diagnostic tests or toxicology screens to evaluate for medical, or medication- or substance-induced causes of depression. These include

  ○ Endocrine: Hypothyroidism, Addison's disease, or Cushing's syndrome

- ○ Neurological: Parkinson's disease, poststroke, dementia, or seizure disorder
- ○ Chronic pain conditions
- ○ Antihypertensives and other cardiac medications, sedatives, anticonvulsants, analgesics, and others[2]

Initial Management

- Overall
  - ○ Evaluate risks for suicide and/or homicide.
  - ○ Evaluate need for hospitalization versus outpatient treatment.
  - ○ Ensure proper diagnosis and treat accordingly.
  - ○ Psychotherapy and pharmacotherapy alone or in combination are effective.[2] This decision can be based upon the severity and type of the depression, and patient preference.
- Bipolar disorder
  - ○ Mood stabilizers are utilized for the acute and maintenance phases.[2,10]
    - Lithium carbonate, valproate, carbamazepine, or lamotrigine
    - Atypical or typical antipsychotics
    - Benzodiazepines: Clonazepam and lorazepam
  - ○ Antidepressants are utilized for bipolar depression and maintenance along with a mood stabilizer.[2]
- Major depressive disorder
  - ○ Psychotherapy options include cognitive behavioral therapy, interpersonal therapy, or psychoanalytically oriented therapy.[2,11,12]
  - ○ Pharmacotherapy recommendations include SSRIs or SNRIs. Selection depends upon factors such as previous treatment response, interactions or contraindications with concurrent medications or illnesses, family history of treatment response, and symptom severity.[2,11]
- Persistent depressive disorder
  - ○ Cognitive behavioral therapy and psychoanalytic therapy are the recommended forms of psychotherapy.[2]

- ○ Pharmacotherapy can include SSRIs, venlafaxine, or bupropion.[13]
- Nonpharmacological recommendations include obtaining proper sleep, stress reduction, exercise, and reduction/elimination of alcohol and other drugs if relevant to the patient.

PERSONALITY DISORDERS

- Personality disorders, or the presence of traits for the disorders, are common and will be seen within a variety of clinical settings. The prevalence of personality disorders ranges from 10% to 20%.[1,2]
- Personality disorders largely involve the use of immature defense mechanisms. These mechanisms are used frequently and become maladaptive ways of coping.[2] See Chapter 4, Patient Education and Counseling, for further discussion on defense mechanisms.

> **CLINICAL PEARL:** Common descriptive terms for personality disorders are enduring or persistent, inflexible, and maladaptive.

- Note that a personality *change* from the individual's baseline (which is more abrupt and not as long-standing as a personality disorder) should prompt a medical evaluation to rule out an organic cause of that symptom.
- Personality disorders are categorized into three clusters (A, B, and C), which share similar features and symptoms (Table 1.3).
  - ○ Cluster A personality disorders are characterized by odd and eccentric behaviors.[1] They include
    - ▪ Paranoid
    - ▪ Schizoid
    - ▪ Schizotypal
  - ○ Cluster B personality disorders are characterized by dramatic, emotional, erratic, and impulsive symptoms.[1] They include
    - ▪ Antisocial
    - ▪ Borderline

TABLE **1.3** Psychiatric History Specific to Complaint

History	Potential Personality Disorder
Distrustful and suspicious	Paranoid
Lacks and does not desire close relationships	Schizoid
Odd, eccentric	Schizotypal
Manipulative, unlawful behaviors, "con man"	Antisocial
Impulsive, unstable relationships, recurrent suicidal gestures or self-mutilating behaviors, splitting	Borderline
Attention seeking, emotional, dramatic	Histrionic
Exaggerated self-importance, need for admiration, entitled, arrogant	Narcissistic
Socially inhibited due to fear of criticism, feelings of inadequacy	Avoidant
Submissive and/or clinging; needs to be taken care of	Dependent
A need for perfectionism and control; not to be confused with OCD	Obsessive-compulsive (personality disorder)

OCD, obsessive-compulsive disorder.

- Histrionic
- Narcissistic
  ○ Cluster C personality disorders are characterized by anxious and fearful symptoms.[1] They include
    - Avoidant
    - Dependent
    - Obsessive-compulsive (personality disorder)

CLINICAL PEARL: You may see personality disorders associated with the terms Mad (Cluster A), Bad (Cluster B), and Sad (Cluster C) to help remember the cluster descriptions. (Note that "mad" is not synonymous with "angry" in this instance, but rather, to be mentally ill.)

Differential Diagnosis

- Another personality disorder within the same cluster
- Depression
- Anxiety

- Psychosis
- Substance use disorder[1,2]

History

CLUSTER **A**
- Paranoid personality disorder symptoms
  - Suspicious of others
  - Doubts loyalty of trustworthiness of others
  - Bears grudges
  - Reluctant to confide in others[1,2]
- Schizoid personality disorder symptoms
  - Does not enjoy close relationships
  - Chooses solitary activities
  - Is emotionally detached or "cold"[1,2]
- Schizotypal personality disorder symptoms
  - Experiences ideas of reference
  - Odd or "magical" thinking and speech
  - Suspicious
  - Inappropriate affect
  - Social anxiety
  - Lacks close friends[1,2]

CLUSTER **B**
- Antisocial personality disorder symptoms
  - Lacks empathy or remorse
  - Violates the rights of others
  - Unlawful, manipulative, or deceitful behaviors
  - Aggressive and reckless[1,2]
- Borderline personality disorder symptoms
  - Impulsive, unstable, and fears abandonment
  - Relationships are usually intense and short-lived
  - Inappropriate anger and/or labile mood
  - Expresses chronic feelings of emptiness[1,2]

> **CLINICAL PEARL:** Suicidal gestures or self-mutilating behaviors, including cutting or burning, can occur frequently in borderline personality disorder.[1,2]

> **CLINICAL PEARL:** Splitting may also occur, in which the patient views others as either all good or all bad. An example of splitting is when you are told you are the only one who can help, and other providers are worthless.[1,2]

- Histrionic personality disorder symptoms
  - Attention-seeking and emotional
  - Seductive or provocative behaviors
  - Dramatic or theatrical actions or speech
  - Easily influenced
  - Considers relationships to be closer than they really are[1,2]
- Narcissistic personality disorder symptoms
  - Grandiose
  - Requires admiration
  - Lacks empathy
  - Boastful
  - Arrogant and entitled
    - Will seek only what he or she perceives is the "best" care.
    - Feels that he or she cannot associate with others who are not at his or her high level.[1,2]

CLUSTER C
- Avoidant personality disorder symptoms
  - Avoids interpersonal contact due to fear of criticism or rejection
  - Unwilling to form relationships due to feelings of inadequacy
  - Reluctant to take risks or join new activities[1,2]

- Dependent personality disorder symptoms
  - ○ Difficulty making decisions without excessive advice or reassurance
  - ○ Difficulty initiating projects
  - ○ Feels uncomfortable or helpless when alone
  - ○ Fears having to take care of self[1,2]
- Obsessive-compulsive personality disorder symptoms
  - ○ Preoccupation with organization, lists, details, rules, and so on
  - ○ Perfectionism that impedes project completion
  - ○ Rigid and stubborn
  - ○ Workaholic; "Type A" personality
  - ○ Holds onto worn items with no sentimental value; "pack rats"
  - ○ Has a miserly spending style
  - ○ Reluctant to delegate tasks; everything has to be done his or her way
  - ○ Rigid moral principles, self-critical[1,2]

Mental Status Examination

The MSE of a patient with a personality disorder will vary depending upon the specific disorder/s. The general appearance may be flamboyant if histrionic or otherwise unremarkable. Speech patterns or phrasing could be odd in schizotypal personality disorder. Mood and affect may be labile if borderline, and angry or charming if antisocial. An anxious mood might be apparent in the avoidant patient. Brief, stress-induced paranoia may occur in borderline personality disorder. Paranoia might also underlie paranoid personality disorder. Otherwise psychotic symptoms are generally absent in the other personality disorders. Insight and judgment are usually poor.

Diagnostic Plan

- Order the appropriate toxicology screens and diagnostic tests to evaluate for comorbid medical conditions.
  - ○ Complete blood count
  - ○ Comprehensive metabolic panel
  - ○ Thyroid function

- Brain imaging
- Others appropriate for specific medical diagnoses

Initial Management

- Psychotherapy is the recommended treatment for personality disorders.[2]
  - Dialectical behavior therapy (DBT) is recommended for borderline personality disorder.
- Medications are not used except to treat target symptoms from other psychiatric comorbidities (depression, anxiety, etc.) that may contribute to impairment.[2]

PSYCHOSIS

Psychotic symptoms are not normal and need to be investigated.[2] Examples of psychotic symptoms include hallucinations, delusions, and disorganized behavior. Hallucinations are false sensory perceptions, so the patient will appear to be responding to stimuli that are not there. Delusions are false beliefs. Disorganized behavior might come from reports of others and/or objective assessment during the evaluation.[1]

Observing or evaluating these symptoms can be overwhelming if you are a novice in your psychiatric training, but the experience can be fascinating as well. Several disorders can present with psychotic symptoms and it is imperative that a proper diagnosis and treatment plan are established.[1,2]

> **CLINICAL PEARL:** Note that temporary psychotic syndromes may occur from anticholinergic, cardiovascular, and steroid drugs, as well as stimulant or depressant medications or illicit substances.[1]

Differential Diagnosis

- Schizophrenia
- Schizophreniform disorder
- Schizoaffective disorder
- Mood disorder (depression or bipolar) with psychotic features

- Brief psychotic disorder
- Substance- or medication-induced psychotic disorder
- Delirium or dementia
- Delusional disorder
- Cluster A personality disorders[1,2]

History

- Patients with psychotic symptoms may not present for treatment willingly and may be brought to attention by others. Psychosocial stressors may be present. The duration of the symptoms is important because several of the disorders have time criteria for diagnosis (Table 1.4).[1]
- As with other common complaints, a past history of prior disorders and treatment is applicable.
- Patients may be experiencing hallucinations but not admit to them because they are frightening to the patient or are recognized as being abnormal.[2]

CLINICAL PEARL: Auditory hallucinations are the most common.

TABLE 1.4 Psychiatric History Specific to Complaint

History	Potential Diagnosis
Psychotic symptoms (hallucinations, delusions, or disorganized behavior) for at least 6 months	Schizophrenia
Psychotic symptoms (hallucinations, delusions, or disorganized behavior) for 1–6 months	Schizophreniform disorder
Psychotic symptoms for <1 month	Brief psychotic disorder
Psychotic symptoms plus a mood disorder	Schizoaffective disorder
Mood disorder causing psychotic symptoms	Mood disorder (depression or bipolar) with psychotic features
Substance, medication, or medical condition	Substance- or medication-induced psychotic disorder
Rapid onset of symptoms (hours to days), which may fluctuate	Delirium
Presence of a nonbizarre delusion without hallucinations or disorganized behavior	Delusional disorder

- You will not want to argue with delusions, nor endorse them during the history-taking process. It is appropriate to ask questions to clarify what is being said, but otherwise challenging delusions is futile.[2]

Mental Status Examination

The general appearance of a patient with psychosis can vary. The patient might be disheveled or more appropriately dressed. Posturing may be seen, which can be a component of catatonia, and involves the patient holding a posture or uncomfortable position for long periods of time. The level of cooperation may vary depending on overall status, paranoia, or level of disorganization. The affect is often flat in patients with schizophrenia. Poverty of speech may be noted. Responding to hallucinations may be observed, such as the patient talking to someone or gesturing to something that is not present. Thought content may include paranoia, delusions, or ideas of reference. The thought process may be disrupted with thought blocking, or include word salad, or incoherence. Insight and judgment might be impaired.

Diagnostic Plan

- Order the appropriate diagnostic tests or toxicology screens to evaluate for medical, or medication- or substance-induced causes of psychosis.
  - Complete blood count
  - Comprehensive metabolic panel
  - Thyroid function
  - Brain imaging
  - Others as appropriate for specific medical diagnoses

Initial Management

- Overall
  - Evaluate risks for suicide and/or homicide in the context of psychosis.
  - Evaluate the need for hospitalization versus outpatient treatment.
  - Ensure proper diagnosis and treat accordingly.

- Antipsychotics are indicated in the treatment of schizophrenia and other psychotic disorders[2,14]
  - First-generation (typical) antipsychotics are dopamine receptor antagonists.[2]
    - These include chlorpromazine and haloperidol, among others.
  - Second-generation (atypical) antipsychotics are serotonin–dopamine antagonists.[2]
    - These include aripiprazole, clozapine, olanzapine, quetiapine, risperidone, and ziprasidone, among others.
    - Clozapine is recommended for treatment-resistant schizophrenia.
- See Chapter 2, Common Disease Entities in Psychiatry, for more information on antipsychotic treatment.

SUBSTANCE USE DISORDER

Substance use disorders affect approximately 7.5% of the U.S. population; affected individuals are all ages and come from various geographical areas and socioeconomic statuses.[15] You will undoubtedly encounter patients with substance use disorder concerns throughout all of your clinical rotations. These concerns may include binge use, intoxication and/or withdrawal, or overdose.

The most commonly used illicit substances are cannabis and amphetamines.[1,2,15] Alcohol, caffeine, and tobacco/nicotine are legal substances that also have high rates of abuse.[1,2,15] Opioids are also commonly abused and can be categorized as illicit substances, such as heroin, or as legal sources such as prescription opioids.[1,2] See Chapter 2, Common Disease Entities in Psychiatry, for a more in-depth review of the various categories of substances.

Differential Diagnosis

- Substance use in the context of conduct disorder or antisocial personality disorder
- Alcohol intoxication and withdrawal is similar to other CNS depressants (sedative, hypnotic, and anxiolytic substances)
- Medical comorbidities mimicking intoxication or withdrawal symptoms[1,2]

History

- Inquire about whether the patient is experiencing symptoms that would meet the diagnostic criteria for substance use disorder: Two or more symptoms over a 12-month period consisting of impaired control of the use, social impairment, risky use, or tolerance/withdrawal.[1] Examples include the inability to cut down on use; craving; job loss or personal conflicts because of the use; driving while intoxicated; signs of tolerance; or withdrawal symptoms such as tremor, nausea, or vomiting (Table 1.5)

TABLE 1.5 Correlating Physical Examination Findings With Potential Diagnoses

Physical Examination[1]	Potential Diagnosis
Slurred speech, incoordination, ataxia, impairment in judgment, attention or memory, stupor or coma	Alcohol intoxication
Diaphoresis, hypertension, tachycardia, hand tremor, vomiting, hallucinations, seizures	Alcohol withdrawal
Restlessness, nervousness, excitement, insomnia, diuresis, GI disturbance	Caffeine intoxication
Headache, fatigue, depression, irritability	Caffeine withdrawal
Conjunctival injection, tachycardia, euphoria, paranoia	Cannabis intoxication
Tremor, diaphoresis, headache, fever or chills	Cannabis withdrawal
Psychotic symptoms, depersonalization or derealization, mydriasis, tachycardia, diaphoresis, tremors; belligerence, violence, or increased tolerance to pain with PCP	Hallucinogen intoxication (no criteria for withdrawal)
Assaultive behaviors, belligerence, dizziness, nystagmus, incoordination, lethargy, blurred vision or diplopia, stupor or coma, euphoria	Inhalant intoxication (no criteria for withdrawal)
Pupillary constriction (pinpoint), slurred speech, drowsiness, respiratory depression, unresponsiveness	Opioid intoxication (or overdose)
Vomiting, diarrhea, lacrimation or rhinorrhea, pupillary dilation, piloerection, diaphoresis, fever, yawning, myalgias	Opioid withdrawal
Euphoria, hypervigilance, midriasis, anxiety, anger, aggressive acting out, cardiac arrhythmias, hyperpyrexia, confusion, seizures	Stimulant intoxication
Fatigue, increased appetite, depression, unpleasant dreams, insomnia, or hypersomnia	Stimulant withdrawal
Anxiety or restlessness, irritability, anger, difficulty concentrating, increased appetite, depressed mood, insomnia	Tobacco/nicotine withdrawal (no intoxication criteria)

GI, gastrointestinal; PCP, phencyclidine.

- The history of a substance use disorder should outline the chronology of the use, route, frequency, and dose, if applicable.

- A history of other substances used is important as well.

- Past attempts at treatment and success should be discussed, as well as complications of intoxication or withdrawal.

- Patients with alcohol use disorder may recall a history of blackouts while intoxicated, or tremor or seizure upon withdrawal. Patients might have gastrointestinal complaints as well.[1,2] CNS depressants such as benzodiazepines or barbiturates resemble alcohol intoxication and withdrawal symptoms.

- Alcohol and CNS depressants cause depressive symptoms during intoxication and anxiety during withdrawal.[1]

- Stimulants/amphetamines can induce psychosis and anxiety during intoxication and depression during withdrawal.[1]

- The history of cannabis use disorder may consist of increased appetite and weight gain during use or sleep disturbance during withdrawal. Respiratory symptoms might be present if cannabis is smoked.[1,2]

- Symptoms of opioid withdrawal may include nausea or vomiting, muscle aches, or insomnia and other objective signs.[1,2]

Mental Status Examination

The MSE of a patient with substance use disorder will vary depending on the substance(s) used. The patient's general appearance may be unremarkable or display signs of intoxication or withdrawal. Patients may appear underweight or unkempt. Some patients appear older than the stated age after years of use. Track marks or other signs of use can be observed. Speech may be unremarkable or slurred during intoxication. Hallucinations can occur during intoxication or withdrawal syndromes. Paranoia, delusions, or signs of disorganization may be present depending upon the substance used. Insight or judgment may be impaired, and the patient might be in denial as to the seriousness of the use.

Diagnostic Plan

- Order the appropriate toxicology screens for substances of abuse and diagnostic tests to evaluate for complications or comorbid medical conditions.

  ○ B12 and folic acid levels

- ○ Complete blood count
- ○ Comprehensive metabolic panel
- ○ Thyroid function tests
- ○ Imaging or other tests as appropriate for specific diagnoses

Initial Management

- Overall
  - ○ Assess the need and patient willingness for inpatient treatment for detoxification or medical comorbidities versus outpatient treatment.[2]
  - ○ Identify and treat overdose/intoxication or withdrawal complications.
  - ○ Psychotherapy and pharmacotherapy options both exist, and are outlined in Chapter 2, Common Disease Entities in Psychiatry, according to the specific substance(s) used.
- Alcohol/CNS depressants
  - ○ A benzodiazepine overdose can be treated with flumazenil, but this does carry a risk of seizures.[2]
  - ○ Acute withdrawal from alcohol or CNS depressants should be treated with benzodiazepines.[1,2]
  - ○ For maintenance treatment of alcohol use disorder, disulfiram, naltrexone, and acamprosate can be used.[1,2]
- Opioids
  - ○ Naloxone, an opioid antagonist, is administered in an opioid overdose.[2,16]
  - ○ Methadone or buprenorphine are commonly utilized in the maintenance treatment of opioid use disorder.[2]
- Tobacco
  - ○ Nicotine replacement using over-the-counter patches, gum, or lozenges is useful.[2]
  - ○ Non-nicotine prescription medications such as bupropion and varenicline can be used as well.[2]

Key Points...

- The most common presentations in psychiatry include depression, anxiety, personality disorders, psychosis, and substance use disorders.

- Certain symptoms can help formulate your differential diagnosis and clue you into a primary diagnosis.

- The MSE is an essential component of the objective patient evaluation, as is a physical examination in other areas of medicine.

- No diagnostic studies exist to confirm psychiatric disorders, but are utilized to rule out other medical causes of psychiatric symptoms.

- Treatments can consist of pharmacological and psychotherapeutic options.

REFERENCES

1. American Psychiatric Association. *Diagnostic and Statistical Manual of Mental Disorders*. 5th ed. Arlington, VA: American Psychiatric Publishing; 2013.
2. Sadock BJ, Sadock VA, Ruiz P. *Kaplan and Sadock's Synopsis of Psychiatry*. 11th ed. Philadelphia, PA: Wolters Kluwer; 2015.
3. Gomez AF, Barthel AL, Hoffmann S. Comparing the efficacy of benzodiazepines and serotonergic anti-depressants for adults with generalized anxiety disorder: a meta-analytic review. *Expert Opin Pharmacother*. 2018;19(8):883–894. doi:10.1080/14656566.2018.1472767
4. Carpenter JK, Andrews LA, Witcraft SM, et al. Cognitive behavioral therapy for anxiety and related disorders: a meta-analysis of randomized placebo-controlled trials. *Depress Anxiety*. 2018;35:502–514. doi:10.1002/da.22728
5. Bighelli I, Castellazzi M, Cipriani A, et al. Antidepressants versus placebo for panic disorder in adults. *Cochrane Database Syst Rev*. 2018;(4):CD010676. doi:10.1002/14651858.CD010676.pub2
6. Pompoli A, Furukawa TA, Imai H, et al. Psychological therapies for panic disorder with or without agoraphobia in adults: a network meta-analysis. *Cochrane Database Syst Rev*. 2016;(4):CD011004. doi:10.1002/14651858.CD011004.pub2

7. Mohatt J, Bennett SM, Walkup J. Treatment of separation, generalized, and social anxiety disorders in youths. *Am J Psychiatry*. 2014;171(7):741–748. doi:10.1176/appi.ajp.2014.13101337

8. Ganasen KA, Stein DJ. Pharmacotherapy of social anxiety disorder. *Curr Top Behav Neurosci*. 2010;2:487–503. https://www.ncbi.nlm.nih.gov/pubmed/21309123

9. Eaton WW, Bienvenu OJ, Miloyan B. Specific phobias. *Lancet Psychiatry*. August 2018;5(8):678–686. doi:10.1016/S2215-0366(18)30169-X

10. Connolly KR, Thase ME. The clinical management of bipolar disorder: a review of evidence-based guidelines. *Prim Care Companion CNS Disord*. 2011;13(4). doi:10.4088/PCC.10r01097

11. Kupfer DJ, Frank E, Phillips ML. Major depressive disorder: new clinical, neurobiological, and treatment perspectives. *Lancet*. 2012; 379(9820):1045–1055. doi:10.1016/S0140-6736(11)60602-8

12. Cuijpers P, Andersson G, Donker T, et al. Psychological treatment of depression: results of a series of meta-analyses. *Nordic J Psychiatry*. 2011;65(6):354–364. doi:10.3109/08039488.2011.596570

13. Levkovitz Y, Tedeschini E, Papakostas GI. Efficacy of antidepressants for dysthymia: a meta-analysis of placebo-controlled randomized trials. *J Clin Psychiatry*. 2011;72(4):509–514. doi:10.4088/JCP.09m05949blu

14. Lally J, MacCabe JH. Antipsychotic medication in schizophrenia: a review. *Br Med Bull*. 2015;114(1):169–179. doi:10.1093/bmb/ldv017

15. Ahrnsbrak R, Bose J, Hedden SL, et al. *Key Substance Use and Mental Health Indicators in the United States: Results from the 2016 National Survey on Drug Use and Health* (HHS Publication No. SMA 17-5044, NSDUH Series H-52). Rockville, MD: Center for Behavioral Health Statistics and Quality, Substance Abuse and Mental Health Services Administration; 2017. https://www.samhsa.gov/data/sites/default/files/NSDUH-FFR1-2016/NSDUH-FFR1-2016.htm

16. Boyer EW. Management of opioid analgesic overdose. *N Eng J Med*. 2012;367(2):146–155. doi:10.1056/NEJMra1202561

ELECTRONIC RESOURCES

Hamilton Anxiety Rating Scale (HAM-A)

> https://dcf.psychiatry.ufl.edu/files/2011/05/HAMILTON-ANXIETY.pdf
> http://www.assessmentpsychology.com/HAM-A.pdf

Panic Disorder Severity Scale (PDSS)

> http://www.goodmedicine.org.uk/files/panic,%20assessment%20pdss.pdf

Yale-Brown Obsessive-Compulsive Scale (YBOCS)

> http://tacanow.org/wp-content/uploads/2013/05/YBOC-Symptom-Checklist.pdf

2

Common Disease Entities
in Psychiatry

Introduction

This chapter reviews common disorders that you will encounter on your psychiatric rotation. Here are a few reminders:

- The etiology of psychiatric disorders is unknown but biological, psychological, and social factors are all suspected to play a role.

- There are no confirmatory diagnostic tests for psychiatric disorders, therefore the *Diagnostic and Statistical Manual of Mental Disorders,* Fifth Edition (*DSM-5*) criteria are utilized in making the diagnosis.[1] A summary of the criteria are included within each diagnosis section given later. Please refer to the *DSM-5* for full diagnostic criteria.

- There are several diagnostic criteria that are common to almost all of the disorders, and these will not be listed for each individual disease listed. These include

  - Impairment in functioning

  - The diagnosis is not better accounted for by another mental disorder

  - The symptoms are not due to a substance, medication, or another medical condition

- Note that impairment in functioning is what separates mental illnesses from "normal" behaviors. Personality traits such as shyness or emotional states such as sadness are not abnormal unless the symptoms are debilitating or interfere with daily activities.

- Various screening tools and rating scales are available to assist in making psychiatric diagnoses. These are described in Chapter 3, Diagnostic Testing.

ANXIETY DISORDERS

GENERALIZED ANXIETY DISORDER

Etiology

Multiple factors are thought to contribute to this and other anxiety disorders. Biological factors include autonomic nervous system disruption, neurotransmitter dysfunction (norepinephrine, serotonin, and gamma-aminobutyric acid [GABA]), or structural or functional brain abnormalities.[1,2] Genetic and familial influences also play a role, as do environmental or social stressors.[1,2]

Epidemiology

The 12-month prevalence of generalized anxiety disorder in the United States is 2.9% in adults and 0.9% among adolescents.[1,2] It is common for other anxiety disorders to co-occur.[2] Females are affected twice as often as males. The age of onset is typically late adolescence or early adulthood.[1,2]

Clinical Presentation

Patients with generalized anxiety disorder experience significant anxiety and worry about a variety of events for at least a 6-month time frame. The worry causes apprehension and is difficult to control. Concomitant physical symptoms are common and include feeling keyed up or restless, feeling on edge, difficulty concentrating, irritability, muscle tension, and sleep disturbance with resulting fatigue.[1,2] Other somatic symptoms such as headaches, nausea, diarrhea, or diaphoresis may occur.[1]

> **CLINICAL PEARL:** Patients may describe having felt anxious for as long as they can remember. They may also be described as a "worry wart."

Diagnostic Criteria

- Anxiety and worry that is generalized (not focused on any one area or phobia)
- Additional symptoms can include
  - Muscle tension
  - Agitation
  - Difficulty concentrating
  - Restlessness
  - Sleep disturbances[1]

Management

- Treatment should include both pharmacological and nonpharmacological components.
- Selective serotonin reuptake inhibitors (SSRIs), buspirone, and the serotonin–norepinephrine receptor inhibitor (SNRI) venlafaxine are recommended, as are benzodiazepines as needed.[2,3]
  - Sometimes patients may be sensitive to the initial activating effect of SSRIs (fluoxetine, in particular) and experience worsened anxiety (especially panic). This effect can be mitigated by prescribing low doses and titrating up slowly.[2]
- Cognitive therapy is recommended, as is behavioral therapy that includes relaxation techniques and biofeedback.[2,4]
- Caffeine and/or other stimulant substances should be reduced or eliminated.
- Exercise has been shown to reduce anxiety.[2]

PANIC DISORDER

Etiology

There is a known familial risk. Serotonergic dysfunction is implicated along with norepinephrine and GABA. Characteristics such as negative affectivity and sensitivity to anxiety may play a role. Smoking is a risk factor. Genetic influences are suspected but not well understood at this time.[1,2]

Epidemiology

The lifetime prevalence is 1% to 4%. The median age at onset is 20 to 24 years. Panic disorder is frequently comorbid with other anxiety disorders, depression, and substance use. As with other anxiety disorders, higher rates occur in females.[1,2]

Clinical Presentation

The intense fear of a panic attack comes on abruptly and is accompanied by physical symptoms. Common symptoms include palpitations, diaphoresis, dyspnea, nausea, or fear of death. The symptoms can abate within minutes to an hour, therefore, this duration can assist in differentiating panic from another medical condition. The attack can occur with no known trigger, such as at night while asleep. Worries about additional attacks will cause patients to alter their behaviors to avoid additional attacks. Individuals with panic disorder seek medical treatment more frequently than those with other anxiety disorders, and may be seen in emergency settings due to concerns that something is physically wrong.[1,2]

Agoraphobia can occur within panic disorder or independently. *Agoraphobia* is defined as a fear or marked anxiety of situations in which escape is difficult, or help might not be available should anxiety/panic develop.[1] Examples include using public transportation, being in either open or enclosed spaces, being in a crowd, or being outside of the home alone in other situations.[1]

> **CLINICAL PEARL:** During a panic attack, patients might express that they feel like they are going to die. This is sometimes characterized by the phrase "feelings of impending doom."

Diagnostic Criteria

- Panic disorder is characterized by ongoing panic attacks.
- A panic attack is an abrupt surge of intense fear or discomfort that peaks within minutes.
- Additional symptoms can include
  - Dyspnea, or experiencing a smothering or choking sensation
  - Chest pain or discomfort
  - Palpitations or tachycardia
  - Diaphoresis
  - Nausea or other gastrointestinal distress
  - Feeling dizzy, unsteady, light-headed, or faint
  - Paresthesias
  - Trembling
  - Fear of dying or "going crazy"[1]
- The patient worries about other attacks or their consequences, and/or changes her or his behavior to cope with the anxiety, usually avoiding potential triggers.[1]

Management

- Treatment of panic disorder includes pharmacological and non-pharmacological modalities.[2]
- All SSRIs are efficacious for panic disorder and are recommended as first-line pharmacological treatment. Specifically, paroxetine is approved by the Food and Drug Administration (FDA) for panic disorder.[5]
  - As noted earlier, patients may experience a worsening of panic after an SSRI is initiated (fluoxetine, in particular). Begin with a low dose and titrate up slowly.[2]
- Benzodiazepines work more rapidly than other medications, but are best used as needed due to concerns with abuse and cognitive impairment. Benzodiazepines can also be utilized short term in bridging therapy while waiting for SSRIs to become effective.

- Regarding psychotherapy, there is no evidence that one form is superior over another, but much research has focused on cognitive behavioral therapy (CBT).[6]

- As with other anxiety disorders, the reduction or elimination of caffeine or other stimulating substances and the addition of exercise should be part of the patient education plan.[2]

SELECTIVE MUTISM

Etiology

High social anxiety or parental social inhibition may play a role.[1] The onset of the disorder may follow an emotional or physical trauma.[2]

Epidemiology

Selective mutism is rare. Prevalence rates are approximately 0.5% to 1%.[2] Social anxiety disorder is a common comorbidity. The onset of the disorder is usually by age 5, although symptoms may not occur until the child is enrolled in school.[1,2]

Clinical Presentation

Children do not initiate conversation or respond when spoken to, despite speaking appropriately and without impairments in other settings. Although they will speak at home in the presence of immediate family members, children with selective mutism may refuse to speak at school, leading to impairment in functioning. Some attempts at nonverbal communication may occur. In addition, they may be willing to engage in activities in which speech is not required. The symptoms should be present for at least 1 month, but not exclusively at the start of school, when taciturn behavior may be considered normal.[1]

Diagnostic Criteria

- Not speaking in situations where speech is expected.
- Ensure that autism spectrum disorder, a communication disorder, or a psychotic disorder has been ruled out.[1]

Management

- Family therapy and education are recommended.
- CBT is recommended as first-line treatment in school-aged children.
- SSRIs can be used as well.[2]

SEPARATION ANXIETY DISORDER

Etiology

At around 1 year of age, separation anxiety can be part of normal development.[1,2] Otherwise, the etiology of the disorder outside of that period is unknown. A significant stressor, such as a death, divorce, move, or change of schools, can trigger its onset. A positive family history can influence the etiology as well.[1]

Epidemiology

Children have higher rates of the disorder but separation anxiety does also occur in adulthood. The 12-month prevalence rates are approximately 4% in children, 1.6% in adolescence, and 1.0% in adulthood.[1,2] The age of onset may occur in preschool through adulthood. There is high comorbidity with other anxiety disorders.[1,2]

> **CLINICAL PEARL:** Separation anxiety disorder is the most prevalent anxiety disorder in children under age 12.[1]

Clinical Presentation

The symptoms will vary depending upon the age of the patient, but overall there is fear/anxiety regarding separation from the home or persons to whom the individual is attached. Patients worry about something bad, even death, happening to their attachment figure(s). Physical symptoms of anxiety may occur along with nightmares, social withdrawal, and apathy.[1,2] The symptoms last for at least 1 month in children or 6 months in adults.[1]

Children and adolescents worry about getting lost or being kidnapped. They fear being alone and may be clingy or follow close behind others, even in the home. Children may have difficulty falling asleep alone and may refuse sleepovers or other overnight stays elsewhere.[1,2]

Adults may be excessively worried about their offspring and/or spouse, especially when separated from them. Disruptions in work or social situations may occur due to the need to continuously check on the whereabouts of a significant other.[1,2]

Diagnostic Criteria

- Excessive fear or anxiety about separation from those to whom the individual is attached.[1]
- Additional symptoms can include
  - Distress over separation from home or from main attachment figures
  - Reluctance or refusal to leave home, sleep away from home, or to go to sleep without being near a major attachment figure
  - Ongoing worry about losing attachment figures or thinking harm will come to them, getting lost or being kidnapped, or being alone at home or other settings[1]
  - Nightmares
  - Physical symptoms such as headache, abdominal pain, or nausea when separation occurs or is anticipated[1]

Management

- Psychotherapy, particularly CBT, is recommended.
- Pharmacotherapy with SSRIs can be utilized as well.
- For moderate to severe cases, both treatments should be combined.[1]

SOCIAL ANXIETY DISORDER (SOCIAL PHOBIA)

Etiology

Genetic and familial influences play a role in the etiology of social anxiety disorder.[1,2] Both adrenergic and dopaminergic dysfunction theories are proposed as well.[2] The onset may follow a stressful or humiliating experience. Behavioral inhibition and fear of negative evaluation are risk factors.[1,2]

Epidemiology

The 12-month prevalence of social anxiety disorder in the United States is approximately 7%.[1] Lifetime prevalence rates range from 3% to 13%.[2] Lower estimates are seen in other parts of the world. The median age of onset is 13 years.[1,2]

Clinical Presentation

Individuals experience inappropriate and persistent fear, anxiety, or avoidance of social situations that involve the potential for scrutiny. Examples such as meeting new people, dining socially, or performance situations (such as giving a speech) cause the individual to worry about negative evaluation, embarrassment, humiliation, rejection, or offending others. The concern is out of proportion to any actual threat.[1] The symptoms should be present for at least 6 months. Self-medicating with alcohol or other substances is common.[1] In children, interaction with adults may be anxiety-provoking and therefore to make the diagnosis in this age group, the anxiety must occur in peer interactions as well.[1] In addition, symptoms in children include tantrums, crying, or clinging.[1]

Diagnostic Criteria

- Persistent distress regarding situations in which the individual may be scrutinized.
- The individual fears embarrassment or humiliation and avoids situations in which this may occur.[1]

Management

- Psychotherapy and pharmacotherapy are recommended.
- Cognitive behavioral psychotherapies are effective for social phobia, and can be used alone or in addition to pharmacotherapy.[2,7]
- Efficacious medications include SSRIs, venlafaxine, or buspirone.[2,8]

- Benzodiazepines or beta-adrenergic receptor antagonists (propranolol, atenolol) can be used as needed in performance-only situations such as public speaking or performing.[2]

SPECIFIC PHOBIA

Etiology

Several psychoanalytic theories have been postulated for the development of specific phobia, but the exact etiology remains unknown.[2] The onset of specific phobia sometimes, but not always, follows a traumatic event. Individuals with negative affect or behavioral inhibition are at increased risk. Other risk factors include parental overprotectiveness, parental loss and separation, and physical and sexual abuse.[1] A positive family history is also seen.[1,2]

Epidemiology

Specific phobia is one of the most common psychiatric disorders.[1,2] The 12-month prevalence in the United States is approximately 7% to 9%. Lower rates are noted in Asian, African, and Latin American countries. As with other anxiety disorders, females are affected more commonly than males.[1,2]

Clinical Presentation

Individuals with specific phobia experience persistent fear, anxiety, or avoidance of specific objects or situations that is out of proportion to the actual harm posed. The phobia is avoided or endured with intense fear or anxiety.[1] Common phobias include animals or insects, heights, water, airplanes, or other enclosed spaces.[1,2] A phobia to needles or blood can also involve vasovagal syncope. Some individuals experience more than one phobia.[1] In children, the symptoms may include crying or tantrums.[1]

Diagnostic Criteria

- Significant fear of a specific object or situation
- Specifiers include
  - Natural environment (heights, water, etc.)

○ Situational (airplanes, enclosed places, etc.)

○ Blood, injection, injury (needles, injury, etc.)

○ Animal (dogs, insects, etc.)

○ Other (for phobias that do not fall into any of the preceding categories)[1]

Management

- The most commonly used behavior therapy is exposure therapy, specifically, systematic desensitization.[2,9]

- Pharmacotherapy options include as-needed use of benzodiazepines or off-label use of beta-adrenergic receptor antagonists such as propranolol or atenolol.[2] The use of SSRIs or SNRIs would be appropriate if another anxiety disorder is comorbid with specific phobia.

REFERENCES

1. American Psychiatric Association. *Diagnostic and Statistical Manual of Mental Disorders*. 5th ed. Arlington, VA: American Psychiatric Publishing; 2013.

2. Sadock BJ, Sadock VA, Ruiz P. *Kaplan and Sadock's Synopsis of Psychiatry*. 11th ed. Philadelphia, PA: Wolters Kluwer; 2015.

3. Gomez AF, Barthel AL, Hoffmann S. Comparing the efficacy of benzodiazepines and serotonergic anti-depressants for adults with generalized anxiety disorder: a meta-analytic review. *Expert Opin Pharmacother*. 2018;19(8):883–894. doi:10.1080/14656566.2018.1472767

4. Carpenter JK, Andrews LA, Witcraft SM, et al. Cognitive behavioral therapy for anxiety and related disorders: a meta-analysis of randomized placebo-controlled trials. *Depress Anxiety*. 2018;35:502–514. doi:10.1002/da.22728

5. Bighelli I, Castellazzi M, Cipriani A, et al. Antidepressants versus placebo for panic disorder in adults. *Cochrane Database Syst Rev*. 2018;(4):CD010676. doi:10.1002/14651858.CD010676.pub2

6. Pompoli A, Furukawa TA, Imai H, et al. Psychological therapies for panic disorder with or without agoraphobia in adults: a network meta-analysis. *Cochrane Database Syst Rev*. 2016;(4):CD011004. doi:10.1002/14651858.CD011004.pub2

7. Mohatt J, Bennett SM, Walkup J. Treatment of separation, generalized, and social anxiety disorders in youths. *Am J Psychiatry*. 2014;171(7):741–748. doi:10.1176/appi.ajp.2014.13101337

8. Ganasen KA, Stein DJ. Pharmacotherapy of social anxiety disorder. *Curr Top Behav Neurosci.* 2010;2:487–503. https://www.ncbi.nlm.nih.gov/pubmed/21309123

9. Eaton WW, Bienvenu OJ, Miloyan B. Specific phobias. *Lancet Psychiatry.* 2018;5(8):678–686. doi:10.1016/S2215-0366(18)30169-X

DISRUPTIVE, IMPULSE CONTROL, AND CONDUCT DISORDERS

CONDUCT DISORDER

Etiology

Risk factors include physical or sexual abuse, exposure to violence, parental rejection and neglect, inconsistent child-rearing practices, strict discipline, frequent change of caregivers, large family size, parental criminality, and association with a delinquent peer group.[1,2] Family history also increases risk. It is interesting to note that a slower resting heart rate as well as autonomic hypofunction have been seen in these patients. Brain abnormalities in frontotemporal–limbic connections have been noted.[1]

Epidemiology

The median 12-month prevalence is 4%. Rates increase through adolescence and are also higher in males, who have a prevalence rate ranging from 6% to 16%.[1,2] Individuals with conduct disorder are at risk for mood, anxiety, psychotic, somatic, and impulse control disorders, as well as posttraumatic stress disorder (PTSD) and substance-related disorders as adults.[1,2] If antisocial behaviors persist beyond age 18, the diagnosis of antisocial personality disorder is made.[1] Comorbidity with attention deficit hyperactivity disorder (ADHD) and learning disorders is common.[1,2]

Clinical Presentation

Individuals generally lack remorse, guilt, and empathy.[1] Males exhibit fighting, stealing, vandalism, and school discipline problems. Females are more likely to exhibit relational aggression and lying, truancy, running away, substance use, and prostitution. Threats or aggression to others or animals/pets is seen. Destruction of property, "conning" others, and theft may also occur.[1] Individuals may suffer consequences in school or at work, legal charges, physical injury, sexually transmitted infections, and unplanned pregnancies. Higher rates of accidents and substance use are seen.[1]

Diagnostic Criteria

- Violation of societal rules or the rights of others
- Additional symptoms may include
  - Destruction of property
  - Deceitfulness or theft
  - Failure to obey rules
  - Aggression to people and animals[1]
- Assess for antisocial personality disorder in individuals whose symptoms persist after age 18[1]

Management

- CBT is recommended.[2,3]
- No medications are approved for use in conduct disorder. Pharmacotherapy with second-generation antipsychotics such as risperidone and mood stabilizers have been studied, but are not recommended as first-line treatment.[2,3]

INTERMITTENT EXPLOSIVE DISORDER

Etiology

Those with a history of physical and emotional trauma in early life have an increased risk, as do those with a positive family history. Dysfunction in serotonin level and the amygdala are also suspected.[1,2]

Epidemiology

The 1-year prevalence rate is approximately 2.7% in the United States. It is more prevalent in younger individuals and in those with no greater than a high school education. Intermittent explosive disorder is also associated with mood, anxiety, and substance use disorders.[1,2]

Clinical Presentation

The primary feature of intermittent explosive disorder is the failure to control aggressive impulses following a stressor that would not normally result in an outburst. The eruptions have a rapid onset and are not premeditated. They typically occur in response to little or no provocation. Less severe verbal or physical episodes occur between more severe destructive and/or assaultive episodes.[1]

Diagnostic Criteria

- Failure to control aggressive impulses resulting in outbursts of behavior
- The outbursts are impulsive and not premeditated
- Symptoms can include
  - Tantrums or verbal arguments
  - Physical aggression toward property, animals, or other individuals
- The aggressiveness is out of proportion to the inciting or precipitating stressors
- The outbursts are not committed to attain something such as money, power, and so on[1]

Management

- Group and family therapies can be helpful. Individual therapy is successful if the patient is willing to work on recognizing and verbalizing thought instead of acting out.[2]
- No one pharmacological agent is recommended or approved. Mood stabilizers/anticonvulsants and antipsychotics have been utilized with mixed results.[2,4] SSRIs, trazodone, and buspirone have also been used to decrease impulsivity and aggressive behaviors.[2]

OPPOSITIONAL DEFIANT DISORDER

Etiology

Oppositional behavior can be developmentally appropriate in early childhood (the "terrible twoss") and adolescence.[2] The disorder is more common in families in which child care has involved a variety of caregivers, or in families who have strict, inconsistent, or neglectful child-rearing practices.[1] Neurobiological factors, such as abnormalities in the prefrontal cortex, the amygdala, and the basal cortisol level, have also been explored.[1]

Epidemiology

The average prevalence estimate is approximately 3.3%, with ranges seen from 2% to 16%.[1,2] Increased rates are seen in males prior to adolescence.[1,2] Symptoms usually appear in preschool-aged children. Common comorbid conditions include ADHD and conduct disorder.[1]

Clinical Presentation

Individuals display ongoing anger; irritability; and argumentative, defiant, or vindictive behaviors. The symptoms may only occur at home. The symptoms need to occur with persons other than siblings because this can be part of normal developmental behavior. Symptoms are more common with parents or others whom the individual knows well. Because it is not uncommon for preschool-aged children to have temper tantrums, the frequency of the behaviors should be noted, as well as whether there is interference in functioning.[1,2] The behaviors should last for a minimum of 6 months.

Diagnostic Criteria

- Symptoms of defiance or vindictiveness, anger, or irritability
- The criteria are not met for disruptive mood dysregulation disorder, and symptoms do not occur during the course of a psychotic, substance use, depressive, or bipolar disorder[1]

Management

- Family therapy is important to develop appropriate management of the child by the parents, and for the therapist to observe parent–child interactions. Structure, appropriate discipline, and consistency are important. Harsh punishments should be reevaluated and support given for positive encouragement by the parents of appropriate child behaviors.[2,5]
- Individual therapy can benefit the child in developing more appropriate behaviors.[2]

- No pharmacotherapies are currently approved for the treatment of oppositional defiant disorder. Some evidence supports the use of risperidone, but it is not recommended as first-line therapy.[5]

> **CLINICAL PEARL:** Kleptomania and pyromania are also included within this diagnostic category. They are uncommon disorders, but the behaviors may occur more often within the context of other disorders such as mania or antisocial personality disorder.[1]

REFERENCES

1. American Psychiatric Association. *Diagnostic and Statistical Manual of Mental Disorders.* 5th ed. Arlington, VA: American Psychiatric Publishing; 2013.
2. Sadock BJ, Sadock VA, Ruiz P. *Kaplan and Sadock's Synopsis of Psychiatry.* 11th ed. Philadelphia, PA: Wolters Kluwer; 2015.
3. Pringsheim T, Hirsch L, Gardner D, Gorman DA. The pharmacological management of oppositional behaviour, conduct problems, and aggression in children and adolescents with attention-deficit hyperactivity disorder, oppositional defiant disorder, and conduct disorder: a systematic review and meta-analysis. Part 2: antipsychotics and traditional mood stabilizers. *Can J Psychiatry.* 2015;60(2):52–61. doi:10.1177/070674371506000203
4. Coccaro EF. Intermittent explosive disorder as a disorder of impulsive aggression for DSM-5. *Am J Psychiatry.* 2012;169(6):577–588. doi:10.1176/appi.ajp.2012.11081259
5. French WP, Kisicki MD. Management of disruptive behavior disorders. *Pediatr Ann.* 2011;40(11):563–568. doi:10.3928/00904481-20111007-07

DISSOCIATIVE DISORDERS

DISSOCIATIVE AMNESIA

Etiology

The etiology is unknown. Adult or childhood traumatic experiences increase the risk for dissociative amnesia.[1,2] Significant acute emotional stress or conflict is an common antecedent in the development of the amnesia.[2]

Epidemiology

The 12-month prevalence in the United States is about 1% to 2%.[1] Other estimates in the general population range from 2% to 6%.[2] No differences are seen between males and females.[2]

Clinical Presentation

Patients will be unable to remember information about themselves; this is not due to normal forgetfulness. The information that is unable to be recalled is usually traumatic or stressful. Dissociative amnesia can include a fugue state, which is travel away from home or bewildered wandering. Some may notice a memory gap or describe "lost time".[1,2]

Diagnostic Criteria

- Inability to remember personal information that is not due to ordinary forgetfulness.
- Medical conditions and substance-induced symptoms have been ruled out.
- Other psychiatric disorders, such as dissociative identity disorder, PTSD, somatic symptom disorder, or neurocognitive disorders, have been ruled out.[1]

Management

- Recommended psychotherapies include cognitive therapy and hypnosis. Group therapy has also been beneficial in retrieving memories of a traumatic nature.[2,3]
- No pharmacotherapies are approved for the treatment of dissociative amnesia.[2]
- If comorbid depression or anxiety is present, it can be treated accordingly.

DISSOCIATIVE IDENTITY DISORDER

Etiology

Dissociative identity disorder is associated with overwhelming experiences, traumatic events, and/or abuse occurring in childhood.[1,2]

Epidemiology

Dissociative identity disorder was previously termed *multiple personality disorder*. Data on prevalence are rare, but estimates on prevalence are approximately 1%.[1,2] Patients are at increased suicide risk.[1]

Clinical Presentation

Patients experience a fragmented identity, with two or more distinct personality states and recurrent episodes of amnesia. They can have intrusions, such as voices, actions, or speech, into their consciousness. The patient may also experience altered affect, behavior, consciousness, memory, perception, cognition, and/or sensorimotor functioning. Medically unexplained neurological symptoms may occur as well.[1] Some cultures may believe this behavior to be possession. Stress often produces transient exacerbation of dissociative symptoms.[1]

Individuals can also experience an altered sense of self or perception such as depersonalization or derealization. Depersonalization occurs when one experiences feelings of unreality, detachment, or being an outside observer of his or her thoughts, feelings, sensations, or body. Derealization is an experience of unreality regarding one's surroundings such as seeming dreamlike, foggy, lifeless, or visually distorted.[1] These symptoms can occur in other conditions, such as panic attacks or PTSD.

Diagnostic Criteria

- The presence of two or more distinct personality states that disrupt the regular identity

- Difficulty remembering personal information, events, and/or trauma that is not due to forgetfulness

- In children, the symptoms are not due to having imaginary friends or other make-believe play, which is considered developmentally appropriate[1]

Management

- Psychotherapy is recommended. Various forms, including psychoanalytic, cognitive behavioral, and self-hypnosis, are recommended[2,3]

- Pharmacotherapy can include antidepressants or medications also used in the treatment of PTSD, including prazosin for nightmares[2]

REFERENCES

1. American Psychiatric Association. *Diagnostic and Statistical Manual of Mental Disorders.* 5th ed. Arlington, VA: American Psychiatric Publishing; 2013.
2. Sadock BJ, Sadock VA, Ruiz P. *Kaplan and Sadock's Synopsis of Psychiatry.* 11th ed. Philadelphia, PA: Wolters Kluwer; 2015.
3. Myrick AC, Webermann AR, Loewenstein RJ, et al. Six-year follow-up of the treatment of patients with dissociative disorders study. *Eur J Psychotraumatol.* 2017;8(1):1–7. doi:10.1080/20008198.2017.1344080

EATING DISORDERS

ANOREXIA NERVOSA

Etiology

The exact etiology is unknown but biological, social, and psychological influences are all implicated.[1-3] Increased levels of cortisol are noted. Risk factors include a positive family history and environmental influences, such as a significant stressor. Children with anxiety or obsessive features are at increased risk. In addition, participation in activities or employment in which thinness is valued places individuals at risk.[1,2] Recent research suggests that gay males are at risk due to expectations and norms for slimness in that community.[2]

Epidemiology

In young females, the 12-month prevalence of anorexia nervosa is approximately 0.5%.[1,2] Males are not commonly affected.

The age of onset is usually during adolescence or early adulthood.[1,2] Depression, social phobia, and obsessive-compulsive disorder (OCD) are frequently comorbid conditions.[1,2] Suicide risk is increased as well.[1]

Clinical Presentation

Individuals with anorexia nervosa experience a distortion in self-perceived weight or shape such that they do not view themselves as others do. Types of anorexia include a restricting type or binge-eating/purging type. Intake can be restricted to only several hundred calories per day due to fear of gaining weight or becoming fat.[1,2,4] Weight loss typically does not alleviate this fear. Patients will engage in behaviors such as excessive exercise and/or use of diuretics and laxatives to prevent weight gain. The individual then maintains a body weight that is below a normal level. Use of the body mass index (BMI) is recommended by the Centers for Disease Control and Prevention (CDC) and the World Health Organization (WHO) as a measure of normal weight.[1] Unusual food behaviors can occur to include hiding food or cutting it into small pieces and moving it around on the plate.[2] Perfectionistic and rigid personality traits are also seen.[1,2]

Significant medical comorbidities can occur as a result of starvation or purging. These include intolerance to cold and potential growth of lanugo, bradycardia, hypotension, amenorrhea, leukopenia, and electrolyte abnormalities, among others.[1,2,4]

Diagnostic Criteria

- Significant low body weight due to limitation of intake
- Lack of insight regarding the severity of low body weight, or experiencing a distorted view of one's body weight or body habitus
- Fear of gaining weight or becoming obese, or participation in behaviors to prevent weight gain[1]

Management

- Most patients resist treatment and are brought for attention by concerned loved ones.

- The treatment of anorexia nervosa involves a multidisciplinary team.[2,3]
  - Individual and family therapy is recommended either on an outpatient or inpatient basis.[2,3]
  - Hospitalization usually is warranted if patients are 20% below expected weight.[2]
  - Involuntary admission may need to be sought if there is a likely risk of death. Inpatient guidelines could involve taking daily weights, measurement of intake and output, restriction of bathroom privileges after meals to avoid purging, and a slow increase in daily calories. Dietitians and medical providers are usually involved in the treatment plan as well.[2,3]
- There are no approved pharmacotherapies for anorexia nervosa. Several medications have been tried with variable results.[2–4]
  - Bupropion is contraindicated due to the increased risk of seizures.
  - Drugs that prolong the QT interval (including tricyclic antidepressants) should be avoided, as fatal arrhythmias can result in the context of hypokalemia.[2]
- Comorbid depression, anxiety, and medical complications should be treated.

BINGE EATING DISORDER

Etiology

Familial/genetic influences may play a role.[1] Extroverted personality traits and impulsive behaviors are associated with binge eating.[2] Stress can induce binge eating as well.[2] Some individuals binge eat to relieve anxiety or dysphoric moods.[2]

Epidemiology

The 12-month prevalence of binge eating disorder among U.S. adults is 1.6% for females and 0.8% for males.[1]

Clinical Presentation

Recurrent episodes of binge eating that occur, on average, weekly for 3 months. *Binge eating* is defined as eating, during a distinct time period, an amount of food that is larger than what most people would eat under similar circumstances. Cultural norms such as eating a large amount during a celebration or holiday meal would not be included in the criteria. The patient lacks control over the binge. He or she might eat more rapidly than normal; eat until uncomfortably full; eat large amounts of food when not feeling hungry; eat alone due to feelings of embarrassment; or feel disgusted with himself or herself, depressed, or guilty afterward.[1]

Individuals with binge eating disorder usually attempt to conceal their behaviors. Binge eating usually occurs as discreetly as possible or while alone. The most common precursor is negative affect but other triggers include stressors, dietary restraint, boredom, and negative feelings related to body weight, body shape, and food.[1]

Patients with binge eating disorder are usually at normal weight, overweight, or obese. It is important to recognize that most obese individuals do not engage in binge eating, and the etiology for obesity (which is not considered a mental illness) is varied, including genetic, physiological, behavioral, and environmental factors.[1]

Diagnostic Criteria

- Recurrent episodes of binge eating
- Associated symptoms may include
  - Overeating despite not feeling hungry, feelings of disgust or embarrassment regarding the overeating, eating at a rapid pace

> **CLINICAL PEARL:** What differentiates binge eating disorder from the binge in bulimia nervosa is that there are no inappropriate compensatory behaviors in binge eating disorder.[1]

Management

- CBT combined with SSRIs is more effective than psychotherapy alone. Exercise combined with CBT is also effective.[2,5] Interpersonal therapy can also be effective.[5]

- There is no one recommended pharmacotherapy agent for binge eating disorder. SSRIs and tricyclic antidepressants can improve mood in those with the disorder. Stimulants are not recommended long term.[2]

- Self-help groups such as Overeaters Anonymous can be effective.[2]
- Fad diets or other quick fixes are not recommended.

> **CLINICAL PEARL:** Pica is the ingestion of nonfood substances, and can occur in the context of conditions such as pregnancy, intellectual disability, autism, or schizophrenia. It can sometimes be attributed to vitamin or mineral deficiencies.[1]

BULIMIA NERVOSA

Etiology

The etiology is unknown. Familial risk and genetic factors may contribute. Biological causes continue to be investigated. Additional risk factors for bulimia nervosa include childhood physical or sexual abuse, low self-esteem, depression, and social anxiety. Social stressors may precipitate the onset as well.[1-4]

Epidemiology

Bulimia is more common than anorexia. The 12-month prevalence rate in young females is approximately 1% but other estimates are as high as 4%.[1,2] The onset is usually in adolescence or early adulthood.[1,2] High rates of bulimia symptoms that are transient and do not progress are seen in young adults.[2] Like anorexia, bulimia nervosa is uncommon in males.

Clinical Presentation

Individuals engage in binge eating and inappropriate actions to avoid weight gain. A binge is consuming an amount of food in a certain period of time that is larger than what most individuals would eat under similar circumstances.[1] The binge-eating episodes usually occur while the patient is alone, but others might notice frequent trips to the bathroom as the individual engages in purging behaviors. Body image or weight is relied upon as an assessment of self-esteem.[1-4]

> **CLINICAL PEARL:** Individuals with bulimia nervosa usually maintain a normal-range weight or are even overweight.

There is a lack of control during the binge during which one feels she or he cannot stop eating.[1] The binge eating and inappropriate behaviors occur at least weekly for a 3-month period on average. Other characteristics include impulsive behaviors and emotional lability.[2] Borderline personality disorder, depression, and substance use disorders may co-occur.[1,2]

> **CLINICAL PEARL:** Vomiting is the most common compensatory behavior to avoid weight gain, but use of diuretics and laxatives also occurs.

Medical comorbidities such as gastrointestinal complaints and electrolyte disturbances are common. Oral complications of vomiting, such as dental caries, chipped teeth, or loss of enamel, can be noted on physical examination. Common electrolyte abnormalities include hypokalemia, hypochloremia, and hyponatremia.[1,4]

Diagnostic Criteria

- Persistent periods of binge eating
- Behaviors to prevent weight gain may include self-induced vomiting, diuretics, laxatives, fasting, or excessive exercise
- The symptoms do not occur only in the context of anorexia nervosa[1]

Management

- Treatment of bulimia nervosa can include psychotherapy and pharmacotherapy. It can usually be accomplished in the outpatient setting.[2]
- CBT is considered first-line treatment.
- SSRIs can play a role in the treatment of bulimia and are usually combined with CBT.[2–4]
  - As noted earlier, bupropion is contraindicated due to its risk of seizures, and drugs that prolong the QT interval should be avoided.

- Electrolyte abnormalities or other medical comorbidities should be evaluated and treated.

REFERENCES

1. American Psychiatric Association. *Diagnostic and Statistical Manual of Mental Disorders.* 5th ed. Arlington, VA: American Psychiatric Publishing; 2013.
2. Sadock BJ, Sadock VA, Ruiz P. *Kaplan and Sadock's Synopsis of Psychiatry.* 11th ed. Philadelphia, PA: Wolters Kluwer; 2015.
3. Harrington B, Jimerson M, Haxton C, Jimerson D. Initial evaluation, diagnosis, and treatment of anorexia nervosa and bulimia nervosa. *Am Fam Physician.* January 1, 2015;91(1):46–52. https://www.aafp.org/afp/2015/0101/p46.html
4. Campbell K, Peebles R. Eating disorders in children and adolescents: state of the art review. *Pediatrics.* 2014;134(3):582–592. doi:10.1542/peds.2014-0194
5. Marly AP, Hay P, Celso Alves dos Santos F, Claudino A. The efficacy of psychological therapies in reducing weight and binge eating in people with bulimia nervosa and binge eating disorder who are overweight or obese-a critical synthesis and meta-analyses. *Nutrients.* 2017;9(3):299. doi:10.3390/nu9030299

GENDER DYSPHORIA

Etiology

The etiology of gender dysphoria is currently unknown.[1] Biological factors such as hormonal dysfunction or genetic causes are under investigation.[2] Psychosocial influences play a role in the formation of gender identity, but it is unknown whether these factors, other than cultural gender norms, are also involved in gender dysphoria.[2]

Epidemiology

The prevalence is less than 1% but is perhaps higher in reality because the data come from only those who seek treatment.[1] Over the past decade, there has been an increase in the number of adolescents seeking care.[3]

Clinical Presentation

Previously known as *gender identity disorder,* gender dysphoria is characterized by distress that occurs when one's assigned (natal) gender does not align with the gender that one experiences or expresses.[1] It is differentiated from nonconformity to stereotypical gender roles. It is also distinguished from transvestic disorder, which involves cross-dressing as a sexual urge or fantasy. Gender dysphoria in childhood does not always persist into adulthood. In other cases, symptoms do not present in childhood but develop at the time of puberty.[1]

Depression and anxiety are common comorbidities.[1] Social relationships and school performance can become impaired due to the stigma that surrounds this disorder.[1,3,4]

> **CLINICAL PEARL:** Children will prefer cross-gender clothing, and stereotypical games and pastimes of the opposite gender.

Some natal boys may pretend not to have a penis and will sit to urinate. Natal girls may refuse to sit while urinating or may express a desire to have a penis. Children will prefer the toys or activities stereotypically engaged in by the other gender and playmates of the other gender.[1]

Adolescents and adults may experience the desire to be rid of one's primary and/or secondary sexual characteristics, and to have the characteristics of the other gender.[1] Adolescents and adults with gender dysphoria are at increased risk for suicide, which may persist even after gender reassignment.[1,3]

Diagnostic Criteria

- Discrepancy between one's natal gender and that which one experiences
- A strong desire to be the other gender
- Associated symptoms may include
  - A strong dislike of one's sexual anatomy, and the desire for the primary and/or secondary sex characteristics of the opposite gender[1]
  - Preference for wearing cross-gender attire[1]

Management

- Current medical recommendations do not involve attempting to reverse the disorder.[1,2] Both the World Professional Association for Transgender Health (WPATH) and the Endocrine Society have standards of care and guidelines that can be referred to.[5,6]

- Parental consent is required for minors seeking treatment.[3]

- Options to suppress puberty include gonadotropin-releasing hormone (GnRH), which can give individuals and families time to further explore other treatments, including hormone administration or surgery.[2] Health maintenance screenings and diagnostic studies are performed to monitor individuals undergoing hormone therapy.[3,4]

- Although psychotherapy is not offered with the goal of reversing the condition, it may be beneficial in coping with the psychological stressors of having the dysphoria, as well as comorbid depression and anxiety.[3,4]

- If comorbid depression and/or anxiety are present, treatment with pharmacotherapy (including SSRIs or SNRIs) for those disorders is appropriate.

REFERENCES

1. American Psychiatric Association. *Diagnostic and Statistical Manual of Mental Disorders.* 5th ed. Arlington, VA: American Psychiatric Publishing; 2013.
2. Sadock BJ, Sadock VA, Ruiz P. *Kaplan and Sadock's Synopsis of Psychiatry.* 11th ed. Philadelphia, PA: Wolters Kluwer; 2015.
3. Vance S, Ehrensaft D, Rosenthal S. Psychological and medical care of gender nonconforming youth. *Pediatrics.* 2014;134(6):1184–1192. doi:10.1542/peds.2014-0772
4. Guss C, Shumer D, Katz-Wise S. Transgender and gender nonconforming adolescent care: psychosocial and medical considerations. *Curr Opin Pediatr.* 2015;27(4):421–426. doi:10.1097/MOP.0000000000000240
5. World Professional Association for Transgender Health. Standards of care. https://www.wpath.org
6. Hembree WC, Cohen-Kettenis PT, Gooren L, et al. Endocrine treatment of gender-dysphoric/gender-incongruent persons: an endocrine society clinical practice guideline. September 2017. https://www.endocrine.org/guidelines-and-clinical-practice/clinical-practice-guidelines/gender-dysphoria-gender-incongruence

MOOD DISORDERS

BIPOLAR DISORDERS

Etiology

The exact etiology of bipolar disorders is complex and not fully understood. Biological, genetic, and psychosocial factors all may contribute. Biological factors include the role of neurotransmitters (norepinephrine, serotonin, and dopamine, among others), hormonal dysregulation (including cortisol), and anatomical issues. Sleep dysfunction and circadian rhythm abnormalities are also hypothesized. A positive family history increases risk. Life stressors and personality factors also play a role.[1,2]

Epidemiology

The lifetime prevalence of bipolar I disorder is approximately 1%.[2] The 12-month prevalence in the United States is 0.6%. The male-to-female ratio is about equal, and the mean age of onset is 18 years.[1]

Clinical Presentation

The category of bipolar disorders includes bipolar I, bipolar II, and cyclothymic disorder.[1]

BIPOLAR I DISORDER

> **CLINICAL PEARL:** Bipolar I disorder must include the presence of a manic episode.

Patients in a manic episode experience an elevated mood described as euphoric or high, but the mood can also be irritable. They will have an increase in energy or goal-directed activities. Grandiose thinking can occur, such as believing that they are someone of importance. This may reach delusional proportions such as thinking that they are the president or have a cure for HIV. Patients with mania require little sleep, are more talkative, and distracted. They become involved in activities with potentially significant consequences such as spending sprees or sexual indiscretions. Impairment should be obvious, and patients may need to be hospitalized.[1,2] A manic episode should last for at least 1 week.[1]

> **CLINICAL PEARL:** The mnemonic DIG FAST can be used to remember the symptoms of mania.
>
> **DIG FAST**
> **D**istractibility
> **I**ndiscretion (in behaviors)
> **G**randiosity
> **F**light of ideas
> **A**gitation and activity increase
> **S**leep decrease
> **T**alkativeness: Pressured speech

BIPOLAR II DISORDER

Bipolar II includes a hypomanic episode and a major depressive episode.[1]

> **CLINICAL PEARL:** A hypomanic episode is similar to a manic episode but does not include psychosis, marked impairment in functioning, or necessitate hospitalization.[1]

CYCLOTHYMIC DISORDER

Cyclothymic disorder is another mood disorder in which chronic fluctuating moods are present, but they do not meet the criteria for major depression, mania, or hypomania.[1]

Diagnostic Criteria—Manic Episode

- Elevated mood (or irritability) and increased energy
- Additional symptoms may include
  - Increased self-esteem or grandiose thinking
  - Pressured speech
  - Flight of ideas or racing thoughts
  - Sleeping little to none
  - Poor judgment and behaviors[1]

- The mania impairs the individual, requires hospitalization, or psychotic features are present[1]

> **CLINICAL PEARL:** Psychotic symptoms can occur in the context of a mood disorder (mania or depression). When this happens, the diagnosis is bipolar disorder with psychotic features, or major depression with psychotic features, and not schizophrenia.

Management

- Evaluate the need for hospitalization if suicide or homicide risk is present, or if the patient is unable to care for himself or herself.

- Treatment is focused on the acute mania and also prevention of further mood episodes.

- Triggers of a manic episode, such as sleep disruption or substance use, should be noted and eliminated if possible.[2]

- Mood stabilizers are indicated for the acute phase of mania or hypomania, and for ongoing maintenance treatment to prevent further mood exacerbations.[2,3] For many patients, the drug used for maintenance is what the patient responded well to in the acute phase.[3] Option include

  ○ Lithium carbonate

  ○ Valproate

  ○ Carbamazepine

  ○ Lamotrigine

  ○ Atypical antipsychotics

> **CLINICAL PEARL:** Lamotrigine carries an uncommon risk of Stevens–Johnson syndrome. Monitor patients and provide education for them to look out for a rash.

- Benzodiazepines can be used short term, in conjunction with mood stabilizers, in acute mania to assist with obtaining a euthymic mood state. Clonazepam and lorazepam are both recommended.[2]

- Antidepressants are utilized in conjunction with mood stabilizers for the depressed phase of bipolar disorder and maintenance therapy.[2]

MAJOR DEPRESSIVE DISORDER

Etiology

Biologic, genetic, and psychosocial elements play a role in the etiology of depression.[1,2] Serotonin is one of the neurotransmitters thought to be implicated. A neurotic temperament and positive family history are risk factors for major depressive disorder (MDD). Environmental factors such as adverse childhood experiences and stressors increase risk. Research has also focused on hypothalamic–pituitary–adrenal axis hyperactivity, genetic variants, and proinflammatory cytokines.[1] Depression is a risk factor for coronary artery disease.[2]

Epidemiology

The lifetime prevalence ranges from 5% to 17%.[2] The 12-month prevalence in the United States is 7% with increased rates in 18- to 29-year-olds compared to those age 60 and older.[1] Overall, there is a higher prevalence in females. Incidence peaks at approximately age 20, but onset is seen in older ages as well.

> **CLINICAL PEARL:** Suicide attempt rates are higher in females, although completion rates are higher in males.[1]

Clinical Presentation

Patients can experience MDD as a single episode or as a recurrent illness. The episodes consist of depressed mood and/or anhedonia that lasts for at least a 2-week time frame. Patients may describe feeling sad, down, or experience somatic symptoms. Additional symptoms include sleep and appetite change, feelings of guilt, and fatigue or decreased energy. Patients might have difficulty concentrating or making minor decisions. Psychomotor agitation or retardation may be exhibited along with suicidal thoughts.

CLINICAL PEARL: The common mnemonic SIG E CAPS can be used to remember the symptoms of a major depressive disorder.

SIG E CAPS
Suicidal thoughts
Interest (loss of); anhedonia
Guilt
Energy (decreased)
Concentration (impaired)
Appetite change
Psychomotor agitation or retardation
Sleep change

MDD and other mood disorders can occur in the peripartum context, in a seasonal pattern, with anxious features, or with psychotic symptoms, among others.[1,2]

It is important to note that depression can present differently in children and the elderly. Children and adolescents may present with irritability, which is noted in the diagnostic criteria. Young children may not be able to express their mood or symptoms but may be observed to be sad or listless.[2] Somatic complaints such as headaches or abdominal pain are common in both children and elderly. Elderly patients may actually deny depression and further probing during history taking may be required.

Diagnostic Criteria

- Depressed mood or anhedonia for a minimum of 2 weeks
- Associated symptoms may include
  - Sleep disturbance
  - Weight or appetite change
  - Low energy or fatigue
  - Difficulty concentrating or making decisions
  - Feeling guilty or worthless
  - Suicidal ideation[1]
- There has never been a manic or hypomanic episode;[1] if so, the diagnosis would be bipolar disorder I (if manic) or II (if hypomanic)

- The Patient Health Questionnaire-9 (PHQ-9) can be used to screen MDD from depression

Management

- Psychotherapy and pharmacotherapy are both recommended, either alone or in combination. In milder forms, either is recommended but in more severe depression, there is much evidence to support a combination of both. This applies to all age ranges.[2,4]
- Psychotherapy options include CBT, interpersonal therapy, or psychoanalytically oriented therapy.[2,4,5]
- Pharmacotherapy recommendations include SSRIs or SNRIs. Selection depends upon factors such as previous treatment response, interactions or contraindications with concurrent medications or illnesses, family history of treatment response, and symptom severity.[2,4]
  - ○ Note that an FDA black-box warning exists for antidepressants, as they may increase the risk of suicidal thinking and behavior in some children and adolescents with MDD. This status is not without controversy, because depression in and of itself increases suicide risk. Current recommendations advise assessing the risk/benefit ratio of use in these age ranges.[2]
- Exercise has been shown to improve depressive symptoms.[2]
- Patient education should focus on decreasing or eliminating comorbid substances that may further contribute to depression, such as alcohol and central nervous system (CNS) depressants[2]

PERSISTENT DEPRESSIVE DISORDER (DYSTHYMIA)

Etiology

The etiology is unknown and likely multifactorial. Biological factors such as neuroendocrine dysfunction and psychosocial influences play a role.[2] Risk factors include childhood parental loss or separation and positive family history.[1]

Epidemiology

This disorder is common, affecting approximately 5% to 6% of the general population.[2] The 12-month prevalence is approximately 1%. As with MDD, females experience higher rates.[1]

Clinical Presentation

Patients with persistent depressive disorder experience chronic depression. They feel depressed most of the time and the duration needs to be at least 2 years to make the diagnosis. The onset is usually insidious and occurs early in life. Individuals commonly have a negative outlook or are pessimistic. Patients may experience increase or decrease in sleep and/or appetite. Lack of energy or fatigue may also be present. Patients may also experience difficulty concentrating and hopelessness. In children and adolescents, the mood can be irritable. Major depressive episodes may precede or occur within persistent depressive disorder.[1,2] Coexisting anxiety or substance use disorders can occur.[2]

> **CLINICAL PEARL:** Most patients with dysthymic disorder report that they have always felt depressed.[1,2]

Diagnostic Criteria

- Chronic depressed mood
- Associated symptoms may include
  - Negative outlook or pessimism
  - Low self-esteem
  - Sleep disturbance
  - Disruption in appetite
  - Fatigue or decreased energy[1]

Management

- A combination of psychotherapy and pharmacotherapy is utilized.
- CBT and psychoanalytic therapy are the recommended forms of psychotherapy.[2]
- Pharmacotherapy can include SSRIs, venlafaxine, or bupropion.[2,6]
- Other patient education points discussed in the Major Depressive Disorder section are relevant for persistent depressive disorder as well.

REFERENCES

1. American Psychiatric Association. *Diagnostic and Statistical Manual of Mental Disorders.* 5th ed. Arlington, VA: American Psychiatric Publishing; 2013.
2. Sadock BJ, Sadock VA, Ruiz P. *Kaplan and Sadock's Synopsis of Psychiatry.* 11th ed. Philadelphia, PA: Wolters Kluwer; 2015.
3. Connolly KR, Thase ME. The clinical management of bipolar disorder: a review of evidence-based guidelines. *Prim Care Companion CNS Disord.* 2011;13(4). doi:10.4088/PCC.10r01097
4. Kupfer DJ, Frank E, Phillips ML. Major depressive disorder: new clinical, neurobiological, and treatment perspectives. *Lancet.* 2012; 379(9820):1045–1055. doi:10.1016/S0140-6736(11)60602-8
5. Cuijpers P, Andersson G, Donker T, van Straten A. Psychological treatment of depression: results of a series of meta-analyses. *Nordic J Psychiatry.* 2011;65(6):354–364. doi:10.3109/08039488.2011.596570
6. Levkovitz Y, Tedeschini E, Papakostas GI. Efficacy of antidepressants for dysthymia: a meta-analysis of placebo-controlled randomized trials. *J Clin Psychiatry.* 2011;72(4):509–514. doi:10.4088/JCP.09m05949blu

NEUROCOGNITIVE DISORDERS

DELIRIUM

Etiology

Delirium is a disorder of cognitive impairment that can be caused by a number of medical conditions, and/or substance intoxication or withdrawal, including prescription drugs.[1] Common examples include

- Cardiac—heart failure, arrhythmias, myocardial infarction
- CNS—seizures, head trauma, brain tumors, or hemorrhages
- Hematological—anemia, leukemia, blood dyscrasias
- Hepatic—hepatitis, cirrhosis, hepatic failure
- Medications—anticholinergic, antihypertensives, antibiotics, opioids, steroids, and some nutritional supplements
- Metabolic or endocrinological disorders—electrolyte, glucose, thyroid, or adrenal dysfunctions

- Pulmonary—hypoxic states, syndrome of inappropriate antidiuretic hormone (SIADH)
- Renal—renal failure/acute kidney injury, uremia
- Systemic disorders—infections, fluid overload or dehydration, neoplasms, nutritional deficiencies
- Toxins—substances of abuse, heavy metals[1]

There are many risk factors for delirium. Common risks include

- Underlying cognitive impairment
- Older age
- Male gender
- Hearing or visual impairment
- Immobility
- Dehydration and/or malnutrition
- Prior history of delirium
- The use of psychoactive or anticholinergic drugs
- Alcohol use disorder
- Other medical comorbidities
- In children, a risk factor is fever[1,2]

Epidemiology

The prevalence of delirium in hospitalized patients is much higher than in the community. Delirium can affect up to half of all hospitalized patients and older patients in the postoperative phase.[2] Approximately 60% of nursing home residents can experience delirium and the rates reach almost 90% in the ICU.[1,2] You may hear *ICU psychosis* used as an alternative term for *delirium*.

Clinical Presentation

The patient will exhibit impairments in attention, awareness, and cognition. He or she may be unable to focus on what you are asking or sustain attention for periods of time. You may need to repeat questions. The individual can also perseverate with an answer to a previous question. Individuals may display mood lability or emotional disturbances that cause him or her to become agitated, call out, yell, and so on. He or she might become easily distracted by stimuli. The patient will likely be disoriented to person, place, and/or time. Memory impairment and perceptual disturbances can also occur.[2]

> **CLINICAL PEARL:** The most common hallucination in dementia and delirium is visual.

Symptoms can worsen in the evening. A disruption in the sleep–wake cycle can also occur. It can range from a mild disturbance in which patients are overly tired during the day and have difficulty falling asleep at night, or a complete reversal in which patients are awake all night and asleep during the day. Finally, a delirium is attributable to an underlying medical condition, substance intoxication or withdrawal, use of a medication, a toxin exposure, or a combination of these factors.[2] The underlying cause should be investigated.

> **CLINICAL PEARL:** The onset of symptoms in delirium is acute; hours to days, for example. This is contrasted with dementia, which usually progresses over a longer period of time.

Diagnostic Criteria

- Altered cognition, attention, or awareness
- The onset is acute
- Symptoms may fluctuate during the day and can include
  - Disorientation
  - Memory impairment
  - Difficulty focusing or paying attention
  - Perceptual disturbances[2]

Management

- The management of delirium is to identify and treat the underlying cause.[1]
- Undetected and untreated delirium can lengthen the duration of the episode and lead to coma or death.[1,2] It is challenging to assess

whether a patient has delirium superimposed upon an underlying dementia, but attempts should be made to do so.

- No one pharmacological agent is recommended, but haloperidol and second-generation (atypical) antipsychotics have been used to treat the psychotic symptoms of the delirium.[1,3,4] These are not without side effects, however. A black-box warning exists for increased risk of death for the use of antipsychotics in patients with dementia.

- Most patients recover, but some symptoms may persist for several months. Some patients do not fully return to a healthy cognitive baseline.

MAJOR NEUROCOGNITIVE DISORDER

Etiology

Major neurocognitive disorder (NCD) is synonymous with dementia. It exists on a spectrum of cognitive impairment. The greatest risk factor is age.[2] Other risks include traumatic brain injury (TBI), genetic susceptibility, metabolic dysfunctions, infections, drugs or other toxins, and cardiovascular disease.[1,2]

> **CLINICAL PEARL:** The most common subtype of dementia/ neurocognitive disorder is Alzheimer's disease.[1,2]

Epidemiology

Prevalence varies by etiological subtype but rates are approximately 1% to 2% at age 65 and reach 30% by age 85.[2]

Clinical Presentation

The presentation will vary depending on the etiological subtype, which is outlined later. Keep in mind that the history may come from the individual or a loved one. The subtypes are classified according to the known or presumed etiology/pathology causing the cognitive decline. Some of the subtypes have common features. Psychotic symptoms such as paranoia or persecutory delusions can occur in moderate to severe stages of Alzheimer's disease, Lewy body disease, and frontotemporal lobar degeneration. Depression is common in Alzheimer's disease and Parkinson's disease. Agitation can be seen in several subtypes, and can be caused by confusion or frustration.[1,2]

Diagnostic Criteria

- Deterioration in cognitive function
- Impairments may be found in
  - Attention, memory, language, executive function, and learning
- Perceptual disturbances may occur
- Instrumental activities of daily living (IADL) are impaired[2]

> **CLINICAL PEARL:** There is a diagnostic category for mild neurocognitive disorder. In this type, there is modest cognitive decline but no impairment in functioning. Note that the patient may make accommodations to account for the decline, however.[2]

Specific etiological types of major NCD/dementia include[2]

- Alzheimer's disease
  - The most common cause of dementia/NCD
  - Insidious onset and gradual progression of symptoms
  - The parietal and temporal areas are affected
  - Impairment in memory and learning is seen early in the course of disease
  - Other early symptoms include depression and/or apathy
  - Moderate symptoms include psychosis, agitation, or wandering
  - Late-stage symptoms include gait disturbance, dysphagia, incontinence, seizures, or myoclonus
  - Mean duration of survival after diagnosis is 10 years[2]

> **CLINICAL PEARL:** Pathological hallmarks of the disease are cortical atrophy, neuritic plaques due to amyloid deposits, and neurofibrillary tangles due to tau deposits.[1,2]

- ○ Genetic testing exists for presenilin 1, which is causative for Alzheimer's disease[2]
- Frontotemporal lobar degeneration (Pick's disease)
  - ○ Insidious onset and gradual progression
  - ○ Symptoms characterized by behavioral or language dysfunction
  - ○ Behavioral symptoms may include
    - Disinhibition
    - Apathy
    - Loss of compassion
    - Changes in eating patterns
    - Compulsive/ritualistic behaviors (such as hoarding)
    - Poor judgment
  - ○ Language deterioration can be noted in speech production or comprehension, word finding, and/or object naming
  - ○ Learning and memory are not as impaired as in Alzheimer's disease
  - ○ Decline is usually faster in comparison to Alzheimer's disease
  - ○ Brain imaging may reveal atrophy in the frontal or temporal lobes[1,2]
- HIV infection
  - ○ Cognitive impairment in the context of HIV infection
  - ○ Symptoms are variable due to HIV affecting multiple areas of the brain[2]
- Huntington disease
  - ○ Cognitive impairment in the context of Huntington disease
  - ○ Insidious onset and gradual progression
  - ○ Symptoms include motor abnormalities, depression, and psychosis[1,2]
- Lewy body disease
  - ○ The third most common cause of dementia/NCD
  - ○ Insidious onset and gradual progression
  - ○ Attention and alertness will fluctuate

- ⊃ Detailed visual hallucinations
- ⊃ Spontaneous symptoms of parkinsonism, with onset at least 1 year *after* the development of cognitive decline[2]

CLINICAL PEARL: The dementia that occurs with Parkinson's disease presents with parkinsonism first, and then cognitive decline. Lewy body dementia presents with cognitive deficits first, and then parkinsonism.

CLINICAL PEARL: Be sure to rule out parkinsonian features as an extrapyramidal side effect of neuroleptic medications.

- ⊃ Symptoms may resemble a delirium
- ⊃ Patients may have rapid eye movement sleep disorder
- ⊃ Depression, delusions, or other hallucinations can also occur
- ⊃ Other potential symptoms include falls, syncope, orthostatic hypotension, and urinary incontinence[2]

CLINICAL PEARL: Patients with Lewy body disease may be sensitive to neuroleptic medications. They may experience side effects to a greater degree, or are at increased risk for neuroleptic malignant syndrome (see Chapter 5, Urgent Management).

- Parkinson's disease
  - ⊃ Insidious onset and gradual progression in the context of Parkinson's disease
  - ⊃ Symptoms include
    - ▪ Apathy, depression, or anxiety
    - ▪ Hallucinations and/or delusions
    - ▪ Personality changes
    - ▪ Rapid eye movement sleep behavior disorder and excessive daytime sleepiness[2]
  - ⊃ To differentiate Parkinson's disease dementia (which involves Lewy bodies) from Lewy body dementia, the Parkinson's symptoms must have occurred *before* (1 year prior to) the cognitive deficits[2]

- Prion disease
  - Onset is insidious and progression of impairment is usually rapid[2]
  - Motor features of prion disease (myoclonus, ataxia, chorea, or dystonia) or biomarker evidence is present[2]
  - Creutzfeldt-Jakob ("mad cow") disease is the most common example of a prion disease[2]
- Substance/medication use
  - Cognitive impairment that persists beyond the time frame of intoxication and acute withdrawal[2]
  - The long-term use of alcohol is a common cause of substance-induced dementia[1,2]
- TBI
  - Evidence of TBI, which may include loss of consciousness, disorientation, amnesia, or other neurological effects
  - Cognitive deficits persist beyond the acute postinjury period
  - Associated symptoms can include personality change, emotional disturbances (anxiety, irritability, lability), or physical symptoms such as headache, fatigue, sleep disruption, vertigo or dizziness, tinnitus or hyperacusis, and photosensitivity[2]
- Vascular disease
  - The second most common cause of dementia/NCD[1,2]
  - The cognitive deficits are associated with a cerebrovascular event/s
  - Cerebrovascular disease is detected upon history, physical examination, and/or neuroimaging[1,2]
  - Symptoms are variable due to the extent of the underlying cerebrovascular disease; for example, an acute infarct versus chronic small vessel ischemic changes
- NCD due to another medical condition
  There may be other causes of NCD that do not fit well into the subtype categories outlined previously. Examples include
  - Structural lesions such as brain tumors, subdural hematoma, hydrocephalus

- ○ Hypoxia
- ○ Endocrine conditions such as hypothyroidism or hypo-glycemia
- ○ Nutritional deficiencies such as thiamine
- ○ Infectious conditions such as neurosyphilis
- ○ Immune disorders such as temporal arteritis or systemic lupus erythematosus
- ○ Hepatic or renal failure
- ○ Metabolic conditions
- ○ Other neurological conditions such as epilepsy or multiple sclerosis[1,2]
- NCD due to multiple etiologies

Finally, a diagnosis of NCD due to multiple etiologies may be used when there is evidence that the patient has more than one medical condition that is contributing to the cognitive decline.[2] See Table 2.1 to differentiate symptoms of the common dementias.

Management

- Accurate diagnosis is essential. A thorough medical diagnostic evaluation should occur. Rule out potentially treatable conditions before coming to a diagnosis of a progressive dementia. Some ill-nesses that are considered "reversible" dementias, such as normal pressure hydrocephalus or hypothyroidism, can be easily detected and should be treated.[1]
- Preventive measures are important for vascular dementia, in which hypertension and other cardiovascular risks should be reduced as much as possible. Diabetes should be kept under control, and the importance of a healthy diet and exercise regimen should be stressed.[1]
- Avoid drugs with anticholinergic properties.[1]
- Cholinesterase inhibitors do not stop the progression of dementia but may slow it in mild to moderate disease. Donepezil is better tolerated than the others in this class.[1,5]
- Memantine can be added to cholinesterase inhibitors and works by reducing glutamate levels, which are thought to have a neurotoxic effect.[1]

TABLE 2.1 Differentiating the Common Dementias

Dementia Subtype	Insidious Onset	Gradual Progression	Memory/Learning Impairment	Attention/ Alertness Impairment	Behavioral/ Language Impairment	Psychosis
Alzheimer	+	+	+			
Lewy body	+	+		+		+
Frontotemporal	+	+			+	
Vascular	+/−	+/−				

- At this time, there is not enough evidence to support the use of supplements such as vitamin E or gingko biloba in the prevention or treatment of dementia. Estrogen replacement and nonsteroidal anti-inflammatory drugs (NSAIDS) also need further study. Mentally and socially stimulating activities may not reduce the risk of dementia, but can be recommended.[1]

- Note that a black-box warning exists regarding the use of antipsychotics in patients with dementia. Antipsychotics are utilized for the neuropsychiatric symptoms of some dementias, such as agitation or psychosis. There was found to be an increased risk of death and cerebrovascular events, including stroke.

REFERENCES

1. Sadock BJ, Sadock VA, Ruiz P. *Kaplan and Sadock's Synopsis of Psychiatry.* 11th ed. Philadelphia, PA: Wolters Kluwer; 2015.
2. American Psychiatric Association. *Diagnostic and Statistical Manual of Mental Disorders.* 5th ed. Arlington, VA: American Psychiatric Publishing; 2013.
3. Hipp DM, Ely EW. Pharmacological and nonpharmacological management of delirium in critically ill patients. *Neurotherapeutics.* 2012;9(1): 158–175. doi:10.1007/s13311-011-0102-9
4. Burry L, Mehta S, Perreault MM, et al. Antipsychotics for treatment of delirium in hospitalised non-ICU patients. *Cochrane Database Syst Rev.* 2018;(6):CD005594. doi:10.1002/14651858.CD005594.pub3
5. Birks JS, Harvey RJ. Donepezil for dementia due to Alzheimer's disease. *Cochrane Database Syst Rev.* 2018;(6):CD001190. doi:10.1002/14651858 .CD001190.pub3

NEURODEVELOPMENTAL DISORDERS

ATTENTION DEFICIT HYPERACTIVITY DISORDER

Etiology

The etiology of ADHD is unknown. Risk is increased with a positive family history. Associations with smoking in pregnancy exist as well.[1] Dopamine and the prefrontal cortex have been the focus of research, as well as maternal infections and prematurity.[2,3] There is no evidence to support that food additives, colorings or preservatives, or sugar contributes to the etiology.[2]

Epidemiology

ADHD occurs in approximately 5% to 8% of children and 2.5% of adults.[1,2] In childhood, ADHD occurs more frequently in males.[1] The onset of symptoms is prior to age 12 per the diagnostic criteria.[1]

Clinical Presentation

Patients with ADHD display symptoms of inattention, disorganization, and/or hyperactivity–impulsivity. Examples of inattention and disorganization can include losing things, not paying attention, making mistakes, becoming easily distracted, and not staying focused.[1,2] Hyperactivity–impulsivity symptoms involve the inability to sit still and/or remain quiet, fidgeting, impatience, and intrusiveness. Patients may talk excessively. They may be described as "on the go" or as if powered by a motor. Delays in language, motor, or social development may also occur. Several symptoms must have been present before age 12 and in at least two different settings, such as home and school.[1,2]

Diagnostic Criteria

- Inattention symptoms may include
    - Poor attention to details or makes careless mistakes
    - Loses focus and/ or is easily distracted
    - Difficulty with sustained attention or concentration
    - Difficulty with organization
    - Forgetful
    - Loses things
    - Does not listen when spoken to
- Hyperactivity and impulsivity symptoms may include
    - Difficulty remaining still; fidgets, squirms, or feels restless
    - Difficulty remaining quiet; talks excessively

- ○ Interrupts or blurts out answers
- ○ Impatient or intrusive
- ○ The Connors and Vanderbilt scales can be utilized in assisting with the diagnosis, and are covered in Chapter 3, Diagnostic Testing[2]

Management

- The first-line treatment for ADHD is pharmacotherapy, specifically stimulants.[2–4]
- Stimulants are contraindicated in those with known cardiac risks/abnormalities.[2,3]
- Nonstimulant options include the norepinephrine reuptake inhibitor atomoxetine, and alpha-agonists clonidine and guanfacine.[2]

AUTISM SPECTRUM DISORDER

Etiology

The etiology is unknown. Familial, genetic, and environmental risks are thought to be involved.[1,2] There is evidence of a heritable risk in families. Genetic abnormalities are suspected and research into these is ongoing.[2,5] Higher incidences are seen with advanced maternal and paternal age, gestational diabetes, first-born children, and perinatal factors that involve hypoxia.[2,5]

Epidemiology

Autism spectrum disorder has a prevalence of approximately 1% worldwide.[1,2] Males have 4 times higher incidence than females.[1,2]

Clinical Presentation

Individuals with autism spectrum disorder display impairments in social communication and interactions in various settings. Symptoms include deficits in social skills and nonverbal communication. Examples include making poor eye contact, difficulty adjusting to appropriate social contexts, difficulty with nonverbal communication, or language impairments. Individuals may also display difficulties with imaginative play, making friends, or lack of interest in peers.[1]

Symptoms also include a cluster of restricted, repetitive behaviors or interests. Examples are lining up toys, difficulty with change in routines, echolalia, inflexibility, distress over change, and abnormal responses to sensory input. Fascination with lights or spinning movements may be present. Motor impairments and self-injury may also occur. Symptoms must be present in the early developmental period. As the name implies, variation in symptom severity is seen along a continuum.[1]

Diagnostic Criteria

- Impairments in social communication and interaction
  - Symptoms may include difficulty in nonverbal communication, social–emotional exchange, and with relationships[1]
- Limited interests or activities, or repetitive patterns of behavior
  - Symptoms may include inflexibility and ritualized behaviors, abnormal reactions to sensory stimuli, and repetitive motor behaviors[1]
- The Modified Checklist for Autism in Toddlers, Revised (M-CHAT-R) can be used to screen for autism

Management

- Treatment for autism spectrum disorders is comprehensive and multidisciplinary.
- Behavioral therapy, educational supports, and parental education and support are all beneficial.[2,5]
- Pharmacological interventions can be used for target symptoms. Risperidone and aripiprazole (second-generation antipsychotics) are FDA approved for irritability in autism spectrum disorder. Research continues into medications for repetitive/stereotypic behaviors and hyperactive/inattentive symptoms[2,6]
- Research into complementary and alternative treatments, such as music therapy, yoga, massage, vitamins, melatonin, and other supplements, is ongoing[2,5]

REFERENCES

1. American Psychiatric Association. *Diagnostic and Statistical Manual of Mental Disorders.* 5th ed. Arlington, VA: American Psychiatric Publishing; 2013.
2. Sadock BJ, Sadock VA, Ruiz P. *Kaplan and Sadock's Synopsis of Psychiatry.* 11th ed. Philadelphia, PA: Wolters Kluwer; 2015.
3. Punja S, Shamseer L, Hartling L, et al. Amphetamines for attention deficit hyperactivity disorder (ADHD) in children and adolescents. *Cochrane Database Syst Rev.* 2016;(2):CD009996. doi:10.1002/14651858 .CD009996.pub2
4. Storebø OJ, Ramstad E, Krogh HB, et al. Methylphenidate for children and adolescents with attention deficit hyperactivity disorder (ADHD). *Cochrane Database Syst Rev.* 2015;(11):CD009885. doi:10.1002/ 14651858.CD009885.pub2
5. Sanchack KE, Thomas CA. Autism spectrum disorder: primary care principles. *Am Fam Physician.* 2016;94(12):972–997. https://www.aafp.org/ afp/2016/1215/p972.html
6. Jesner OS, Aref-Adib M, Coren E. Risperidone for autism spectrum disorder. *Cochrane Database Syst Rev.* 2007;(1):CD005040. doi:10 .1002/14651858.CD005040.pub2

OBSESSIVE-COMPULSIVE AND RELATED DISORDERS

BODY DYSMORPHIC DISORDER

Etiology

The disorder is associated with high rates of childhood neglect and abuse. Risk is elevated in those with a positive family history of OCD.[1] Serotonin dysfunction may place a role.[2]

Epidemiology

The prevalence is approximately 2% in the United States and higher in patients seeking dermatological, cosmetic, and oral–maxillary surgery. The median age of onset is 15 years.[1] Females are affected slightly more than males.[2] The disorder is associated with comorbid anxiety, social avoidance, depressed mood, neuroticism, perfectionism, and low self-esteem.[1] Suicide risk is also higher.[1]

Clinical Presentation

Individuals with body dysmorphic disorder feel that there is a defect or flaw/s in their physical appearance. This is either not noticeable by others or, if present, is slight. They may believe they look ugly, unattractive, abnormal, or deformed.[1] They may have ideas of reference, that make them feel others are looking at or mocking them. Any bodily location can be affected, but the most common areas are the skin, the hair, and the nose. Perceived asymmetry can also be a concern.[1]

The patient will perform repetitive thoughts or behaviors in order to decrease the anxiety over the flaw. Common behaviors include comparing appearances with others, frequent checking or examining of the defect(s) in the mirror, excessive grooming (combing, shaving, styling), camouflaging, seeking reassurance, skin picking, excessively exercising or weight lifting, and seeking cosmetic procedures. Some may tan excessively or change clothing frequently. The thoughts or behaviors are unwelcome, time-consuming (3–8 hours per day), and usually difficult to resist or control.[1]

Diagnostic Criteria

- Fixation on a defect in appearance that is not apparent to others, or if so, it is slight
- Symptoms may include
  - Unnecessary grooming, frequent checking of the appearance in a mirror or other reflective surface, or seeking reassurance[1]

Management

- Treatment should focus on the underlying disorder, and not on the perceived defects. Patients who seek surgical, dermatological, or other procedures to fix any defects will typically develop a new area to focus on.[2]
- CBT is recommended.[3]
- The use of SSRIs or clomipramine has demonstrated a reduction in symptoms.[2,3]
- Comorbid depression or anxiety should be treated as well.[2]

OBSESSIVE-COMPULSIVE DISORDER (OCD)

Etiology

The etiology of OCD is unknown. Familial transmission and genetic factors have been implicated.[1,2] Dysfunction of the serotonergic system is suspected.[2] Increased risk has also been noted in those with childhood physical and sexual abuse and other traumatic or stressful events.[1]

Epidemiology

The lifetime prevalence of OCD in the general population is 2% to 3%.[2,4] The 12-month prevalence in the United States is 1.2%.[1] In childhood, males are slightly more affected but in adulthood the opposite is true. The mean age of onset is approximately 20 years, and symptoms usually begin gradually.[2] OCD is often comorbid with other anxiety disorders, major depression, and alcohol use disorder.[1,2]

Clinical Presentation

Patients with OCD experience obsessions and perform compulsive behaviors to decrease the anxiety associated with the obsession. Obsessions are defined as recurrent, persistent, and intrusive thoughts, urges, or images.[1,2] Compulsions are repetitive behaviors or mental acts performed in response to an obsession or according to rules that must be applied rigidly.[1,2]

Common symptom patterns include contamination or cleaning, symmetry, pathological doubt, and forbidden thoughts.[1,2] Patients with contamination symptoms fear that their hands will get dirty or come in contact with microbes. Pathological doubt revolves around whether something was turned off, unplugged, and so on. Many hours of the day can be spent performing compulsions.[1,2] Patients with OCD may have an inflated sense of responsibility, perfectionism, and the need to control thoughts.[1]

> **CLINICAL PEARL:** Ask patients whether they regularly count, check, or clean things to screen for obsessive-compulsive disorder (OCD).

Diagnostic Criteria

- Obsessive symptoms include
  - Intrusive thoughts or images that are anxiety-provoking[1]
- Compulsive symptoms include
  - Handwashing, counting, repeating words silently, or checking[1]
- The compulsions are performed in an attempt to prevent or reduce anxiety
- More than 1 hour per day is taken up by the obsessions or compulsions[1]

Management

- The treatment of OCD consists of pharmacotherapy and behavior therapy
- The SSRIs or clomipramine are recommended first-line medications[2,4]
- Behavior therapy is effective but some patients may resist treatment[2,4]

Other Related Disorders

- *Excoriation disorder*
  - Recurrent picking of one's skin
  - The most common sites are the face, arms, and hands, but multiple body sites are common as well
  - Individuals may pick at healthy skin, lesions, or minor irregularities[1]
- *Hoarding*
  - Distress over discarding or parting with possessions
  - There is a need to save items regardless of their actual value
  - Clutter and congestion occur in the living areas[1]
- *Trichotillomania*
  - Hair pulling resulting in hair loss
  - The most common sites are the scalp, eyebrows, and eyelids[1]

References

1. American Psychiatric Association. *Diagnostic and Statistical Manual of Mental Disorders*. 5th ed. Arlington, VA: American Psychiatric Publishing; 2013.
2. Sadock BJ, Sadock VA, Ruiz P. *Kaplan and Sadock's Synopsis of Psychiatry*. 11th ed. Philadelphia, PA: Wolters Kluwer; 2015.
3. Ipser JC, Sander C, Stein DJ. Pharmacotherapy and psychotherapy for body dysmorphic disorder. *Cochrane Database Syst Rev.* 2009;(1):CD005332. doi:10.1002/14651858.CD005332.pub2
4. Pittenger C, Bloch MH. Pharmacological treatment of obsessive-compulsive disorder. *Psychiatr Clin North Am.* 2014;37(3):375–391. doi:10.1016/j.psc.2014.05.006

Personality Disorders

Etiology

The exact etiology is unknown. Familial and genetic risks have been noted. Environmental influences may play a role as well. Biological factors such as the role of neurotransmitters or hormones continue to be explored.[1,2] The use of defense mechanisms in personality disorders must also be appreciated.[2]

Schizoid and schizotypal personality disorders may be more prevalent in those with a positive family history of schizophrenia.[1] Risks for antisocial personality disorder include child abuse, unstable parenting, or inconsistent discipline.[1] Patients with borderline personality disorder often have histories of physical and sexual abuse, neglect, early parental loss, and hostile conflict.[1] A history of harsh discipline is seen in patients with obsessive-compulsive personality disorder.[2]

Epidemiology

Personality disorders are common. Approximately 15% of U.S. adults have at least one personality disorder.[1] The symptoms will be recognizable in adolescence or early adulthood and will be chronic.[1] Upward of 50% of patients with another psychiatric disorder also have a personality disorder.[2] Borderline, histrionic, and dependent personality disorders are diagnosed more frequently in females. Antisocial personality disorder is diagnosed more frequently in males.[1]

Clinical Presentation

Most patients with personality disorders will not present with a complaint regarding their personality. This is because the thoughts and behaviors are ego-syntonic; they are acceptable to the ego and do not cause distress for the patient, despite negatively affecting others. They will have limited to no insight into their behavior and might be brought for evaluation by a family member, or may present on their own with a comorbid psychiatric complaint such as depression or anxiety. Consequences of their behavior, such as a job loss or ending of a relationship, might also prompt an evaluation.

Personality disorders are categorized into three clusters: A, B, and C. The clusters share similar features and symptoms. Cluster A is characterized by patients who are odd or eccentric and includes paranoid, schizoid, and schizotypal personality disorders. Cluster B is described as dramatic, emotional, or erratic. Cluster B includes antisocial, borderline, histrionic, and narcissistic personality disorders. Cluster C symptoms are anxious or fearful and include avoidant, dependent, and obsessive-compulsive personality disorders. Finally, patients may present with co-occurring personality disorders.[1-3]

> **CLINICAL PEARL:** You might see the clusters referred to as "mad" (Cluster A), " bad" (Cluster B), and "sad" (Cluster C).

CLUSTER A

- **Paranoid personality disorder** presents with mistrust and suspiciousness. Despite any lack of evidence, individuals feel that others will exploit, harm, or deceive them. They will be reluctant to confide in others and often bear grudges.[1] Patients with paranoid personality disorder generally do not get along well with others, although they may become part of a group that shares common paranoid beliefs.[1] They are often guarded and secretive, and may also be argumentative or aloof.

- **Schizoid personality disorder** is characterized by disinterest in relationships and a restricted range of emotional expression.[1] Patients with schizoid personality disorder will appear cold and aloof. They will have few friends and are often unmarried. They may be employed in positions with little contact with others, or prefer the night shift, for example.[2] They are not likely to seek medical care, but if so, they may appear uncomfortable and display poor eye contact.

> **CLINICAL PEARL:** Those with schizoid personality disorder are "loners" and prefer it that way. This is in contrast to avoidant personality disorder discussed later, in which individuals do not wish to be alone.

- **Schizotypal personality disorder** is characterized by discomfort in close relationships, cognitive or perceptual distortions, and eccentric behavior. Patients will be noticeably odd or strange, and are uncomfortable relating to others. Taking a history might be difficult. Individuals may exhibit ideas of reference, feel that they have magical control, or claim to have special powers such as sensing the future or reading minds. Speech may be unusual and/or vague. They may also display paranoia, especially under stress[1]
  - ○ Patients with schizotypal personality disorder are at risk for developing schizophrenia.[2]

CLUSTER B

- **Antisocial personality disorder** exhibits a disregard for the rights of others. Referred to as *psychopaths* or *sociopaths*, individuals generally lack empathy and are deceitful and manipulative. They will repeatedly engage in activities that are grounds for arrest, and can be aggressive and reckless. They may display inflated self-esteem and can also be charming. Histories of truancy, thefts, fights, and comorbid substance use are common[1,2]
  - ○ The diagnosis of antisocial personality disorder is not given to individuals younger than 18 years and is given only if there is a history of some symptoms of conduct disorder before age 15 years.[1]
  - ○ Antisocial personality disorder is associated with alcohol use disorder.[1,2]
  - ○ Abnormal EEGs and other neurological soft signs indicative of minimal brain damage are sometimes seen.[2]

- **Borderline personality disorder** is characterized by impulsivity and instability in relationships, self-image, and affect. Individuals are often in a state of crisis and will have labile moods. Patients fear abandonment and can display angry outbursts. They may obtain comfort from transitional objects (pets, stuffed animals, or other inanimate objects) and bring them into the hospital or to appointments.[1,2]

  ○ Be aware of splitting, which is when staff are viewed as either all good or no good; these patients either idealize or devalue others, which can be disruptive, especially on an inpatient unit. As a student, you may become an unwilling participant in the patient's attempt to split staff.[2]

CLINICAL PEARL: Self-mutilating behaviors, such as cutting or burning, and suicidal behaviors are common.[1,2]

- **Histrionic personality disorder** is characterized by attention-seeking behaviors and excessive emotionality. Individuals like to be the center of attention and may be lively, dramatic, or flirtatious. Behaviors are exaggerated, and child-like temper tantrums may occur. Patients often consider relationships to be more intimate than they are. They become bored with a usual routine, project, or relationship[1]

  ○ There is a strong association between histrionic personality disorder and somatic symptom disorders.

- **Narcissistic personality disorder** exhibits grandiosity, a need for admiration, and a dearth of empathy. Individuals feel that they are superior to others and tend to boast about their abilities or accomplishments. They may be preoccupied with success, power, or beauty, and require excessive admiration.[1] They may also be sensitive to criticism or defeat, and have an underlying fragile state of self-esteem.[1,2]

CLUSTER C

- **Avoidant personality disorder** is characterized by inhibition, feeling inadequate, and sensitivity to criticism. Patients feel inferior and are timid. Individuals may be shy or quiet in an attempt to remain invisible, and will avoid forming relationships for fear of criticism, disapproval, or rejection.[1] They will rarely speak up in public settings and are often employed in vocations in which they can remain on the periphery. A history of social phobia is common.[1,2]

> CLINICAL PEARL: In contrast to schizoid personality disorder, those with avoidant personality disorder are alone, but do not prefer it this way and need much reassurance of acceptance.

- **Dependent personality disorder** includes a pattern of submissive and clinging behavior related to an excessive need to be taken care of or fear of separation. Individuals feel that they cannot function without the help of others and have great difficulty making simple decisions. They are often pessimistic and filled with self-doubt, and may even seek dominance or overprotection to avoid being alone.[1] Individuals will avoid leadership positions or become anxious if asked to take such a position.[2]

- **Obsessive-compulsive personality disorder** is a pattern of preoccupation with orderliness, perfectionism, and control.[1] Do not be confused by the nomenclature; this personality disorder is different from OCD, discussed earlier.

Much attention is paid to details, lists, rules, and schedules. Individuals will have high standards and may spend excessive amounts of time on tasks. They may be conscientious and inflexible, stingy, and stubborn. They may have difficulty discarding objects, becoming a "pack rat." There is similarity to "type A" personality traits in that those with this personality disorder display excessive devotion to work and productivity, time urgency, and competitiveness.[1]

Diagnostic Criteria

- A long-lasting pattern of internal experience and behavior that differs significantly from cultural norms
- The symptoms are manifested in interpersonal relationships, cognition, affect, or impulse control
- The behaviors are persistent in a variety of situations
- The behaviors are long-standing; the onset can be traced back at least to adolescence or early adulthood[1]

Management

- Psychotherapy is the recommended treatment for most personality disorders.[2–4]

  - Dialectical behavior therapy (DBT) is recommended for borderline personality disorder.[2]

  - Patients with antisocial personality disorder may not respond as well to therapy, and may be involved with the legal system due to their criminal behaviors.[2]

  - Avoidant personality disorder may benefit from assertiveness therapy.[2]

  - Those with obsessive-compulsive personality disorder may be more open to treatment in comparison to the other personality disorders, as they are more aware of their impairments.[2]

- Medications cannot be utilized in the treatment of personality dysfunction, but treating symptoms such as mood lability, depression, or anxiety is appropriate.[2,3] For example, using mood stabilizers for patients with borderline or antisocial personality disorder can assist in decreasing impulsive or aggressive behaviors. The use of SSRIs would be appropriate for the anxious features of Cluster C disorders. Antipsychotics may be utilized for Cluster A disorders or for mood stabilization in Cluster B.

References

1. American Psychiatric Association. *Diagnostic and Statistical Manual of Mental Disorders.* 5th ed. Arlington, VA: American Psychiatric Publishing; 2013.
2. Sadock BJ, Sadock VA, Ruiz P. *Kaplan and Sadock's Synopsis of Psychiatry.* 11th ed. Philadelphia, PA: Wolters Kluwer; 2015.
3. Angstman KB, Rasmussen NH. Personality disorders: review and clinical application in daily practice. *Am Fam Physician.* December 1, 2011;84(11):1253–1260. https://www.aafp.org/afp/2011/1201/p1253.html
4. Carsky M. Supportive psychoanalytic therapy for personality disorders. *Psychotherapy.* 2013;50(3):443–448. doi:10.1037/a0032156

Psychotic Disorders

Brief Psychotic Disorder

Etiology

The etiology is unknown. Risk factors include schizotypal and borderline personality disorder, and those with traits of suspiciousness.[1] Significant psychosocial stressors also pay a role in precipitating the illness.[2]

Epidemiology

Brief psychotic disorder accounts for 9% of new-onset psychosis.[1] Females more commonly experience this disorder.[1] The age of onset is typically in young adulthood to middle age.[3]

Clinical Presentation

The patient experiences at least one symptom of psychosis, including delusions, hallucinations, or disorganized speech or behavior (see Introduction: The Approach to the Patient in Psychiatry). The onset of symptoms is usually sudden, occurring within approximately 2 weeks prior to which the patient had been previously nonpsychotic. The disturbance lasts at least 1 day but less than 1 month, and the individual eventually has a full return to the premorbid level of functioning. Confusion or emotional turmoil is a common symptom.[1]

Diagnostic Criteria

- Presence of hallucinations, delusions, or disorganized speech
- Disorganized behavior or catatonia can also occur, but are not one of the required symptoms for diagnosis
- The symptoms last between 1 day and 1 month, and the patient recovers to the previous level of functioning[1]

Management

- Antipsychotics are appropriate. Benzodiazepines can also be used in the short-term treatment of psychosis.[2,3]

- Medications should be tapered and discontinued after a period of stability is achieved.

  - If the patient's symptoms return, the diagnosis needs to be reconsidered to include schizophreniform disorder or other psychotic illnesses that persist beyond 1 month.[2]

- Psychotherapy can play a role in exploring any stressors that precipitated the event, and improving coping skills.[2]

DELUSIONAL DISORDER

Etiology

The etiology of delusional disorder is unknown. There is a significant familial relationship with delusional disorder and both schizophrenia and schizotypal personality disorder.[1] Advanced age and sensory impairment are risk factors, as is social isolation.[2]

Epidemiology

The lifetime prevalence of delusional disorder is approximately 0.2%. It is less common than schizophrenia. The most frequent subtypes are persecutory and erotomanic.[1,2]

Clinical Presentation

Patients with delusional disorder experience at least one delusion that persists beyond 1 month. *Delusions* are defined as fixed beliefs that are not amenable to change despite evidence to the contrary. The delusional subtypes are listed later. Individuals may admit that others view their beliefs as irrational, but they are unable to accept this themselves. Other characteristic symptoms of schizophrenia are absent.[1]

Diagnostic Criteria

- One or more delusions that have lasted for at least 1 month

- The patient has not met criteria for the diagnosis of schizophrenia

- Apart from the delusion, behavior is not unusual or odd[1]

Subtypes

- Erotomanic type
  - The belief that another person is in love with him or her.
- Grandiose type
  - The belief that one has a great talent or insight, or has made a significant discovery.
- Jealous type
  - The belief that one's significant other is adulterous.
- Persecutory type
  - The belief that one is being watched, followed, harassed, cheated on, slandered, or poisoned or drugged.[1]

> **CLINICAL PEARL:** The persecutory type is the most common type of delusion.[1]

- Somatic type
  - The theme involves bodily functions or sensations.[1] Common symptoms include thinking that one has a parasitic infection or insect infestation on the skin.[1] Sometimes patients will believe they are pregnant, despite evidence to the contrary.

Management

• The treatment of delusional disorder consists of psychotherapy and antipsychotic medications. See further discussion on antipsychotics in the following section on schizophrenia.[2,4]

SCHIZOPHRENIA

Etiology

The etiology of schizophrenia is unknown. Genetic factors are suspected, as a higher incidence is seen among family members with the illness. Dopamine and potentially other neurotransmitters are hypothesized to play a role.[1,2] Other potential risk factors include season of birth, complications of pregnancy or birth, viral illnesses, advanced paternal age, and urban environments.[2] Schizotypal or paranoid personality disorder may sometimes precede the onset of schizophrenia.[1]

Epidemiology

The lifetime prevalence of schizophrenia is approximately 0.3% to 1%.[1,2] The onset of symptoms usually occurs between the late teens and mid-30s. Schizophrenia can occur in childhood but it is rare.[1] Although there is no gender prevalence, symptom onset is typically earlier in males.[2]

> **CLINICAL PEARL:** Elderly patients with new-onset psychotic symptoms should be evaluated for a delirium or another medical cause. It is unlikely that a psychiatric etiology would present in later life.

Clinical Presentation

Schizophrenia is a heterogeneous disorder and no one symptom is pathognomonic. The patient will present with several positive and negative symptoms. Positive symptoms refer to hallucinations, delusions, and disorganized speech, behavior, or catatonia. Negative symptoms include diminished emotional expression (flat affect), avolition, alogia, anhedonia, and asociality.[1,2]

Avolition is difficulty initiating or maintaining activity. Alogia, also called *poverty of speech*, is a reduced speech output in which the patient says very little or hardly offers spontaneous speech. Asociality is the lack of engagement in social interaction and/or the preference for solitary activities.[2]

A prodrome is sometimes seen during the development of the illness, which is characterized by negative symptoms resembling depression. The symptoms need to be present for at least 6 months, which can include a prodrome and residual symptoms.[1] Finally, individuals with schizophrenia have high comorbidity with tobacco use disorder. It is theorized that abnormalities in nicotinic receptors provide a therapeutic effect on the symptoms.[1,2]

CLINICAL PEARL: Delusions of thought insertion or thought withdrawal occur more often in patients with schizophrenia.
Thought insertion is the belief that others are putting thoughts in one's head.
Thought withdrawal is the belief that thoughts are being taken out of one's head.
Thought broadcasting is another delusional belief that the patient's thoughts are being heard by others.[2]

Diagnostic Criteria

- At least one of the symptoms must be hallucinations, delusions, or disorganized speech[1]
- The patient might also exhibit disorganized behavior, catatonia, or negative symptoms[1]
- The level of functioning is below that which was achieved prior to the onset of symptoms[1]

SCHIZOAFFECTIVE DISORDER

This disorder is diagnosed when the patient meets criteria for schizophrenia, and experiences a major depressive or manic episode concurrently.

CLINICAL PEARL: You should distinguish schizoaffective disorder from depression or mania with psychotic symptoms. In schizoaffective disorder, the psychotic symptoms will still be present if the mood symptoms have resolved. A psychosis that occurs secondary to a major depressive or manic episode will resolve along with mood symptoms.

SCHIZOPHRENIFORM DISORDER

This disorder is diagnosed when the symptom criteria for schizophrenia have been met, but the episode lasts between 1 and 6 months. If the duration is less than 6 months and the patient has not yet recovered, a provisional diagnosis of schizophreniform disorder is given.[1]

- As mentioned earlier, if the illness persists beyond 6 months, a diagnosis of schizophrenia is then given.

Management

- Antipsychotics are indicated in the treatment of schizophrenia. Atypical antipsychotics carry less risk of extrapyramidal side effects than the typical class, and are therefore first-line treatment[2,5]

  ○ First-generation (typical) antipsychotics are dopamine receptor antagonists.[2]

    ▪ These include chlorpromazine and haloperidol among others

    ▪ Effective for the positive symptoms of schizophrenia.

  ○ Second-generation (atypical) antipsychotics are serotonin dopamine antagonists.[2]

    ▪ These include aripiprazole, clozapine, olanzapine, quetiapine, risperidone, and ziprasidone, among others

    ▪ Effective for the positive and negative symptoms of schizophrenia

    ▪ Clozapine is recommended for treatment-resistant schizophrenia

CLINICAL PEARL: Clozapine carries a risk of agranulocytosis, and monitoring of white blood cell and absolute neutrophil count is mandated.[6]

    ▪ Atypical antipsychotics can impair insulin metabolism
      - BMI, glucose, and lipid monitoring should occur[2,5]
- Noncompliance is common.

  ○ Long-acting injectable antipsychotics can be used to increase compliance.
- Extrapyramidal side effects should be monitored, including tardive dyskinesia, dystonic reaction, parkinsonism, or akathisia

  ○ The Abnormal Involuntary Movement Scale (AIMS) is used to monitor for tardive dyskinesia. See Chapter 3, Diagnostic Testing, for more information.
- Psychosocial therapy interventions are also recommended.

- If command auditory hallucinations are present (voices telling the patient to do something), evaluate for safety concerns if the command is to hurt or kill oneself or others.[2]

REFERENCES

1. American Psychiatric Association. *Diagnostic and Statistical Manual of Mental Disorders.* 5th ed. Arlington, VA: American Psychiatric Publishing; 2013.
2. Sadock BJ, Sadock VA, Ruiz P. *Kaplan and Sadock's Synopsis of Psychiatry.* 11th ed. Philadelphia, PA: Wolters Kluwer; 2015.
3. Correll CU, Smith CW, Auther AM, et al. Predictors of remission, schizophrenia, and bipolar disorder in adolescents with brief psychotic disorder or psychotic disorder not otherwise specified considered at very high risk for schizophrenia. *J Child Adolesc Psychopharmacol.* 2008;18(5):475–490. doi:10.1089/cap.2007.110
4. Skelton M, Khokhar WA, Thacker SP. Treatments for delusional disorder. *Cochrane Database Syst Rev.* 2015;(5):CD009785. doi:10.1002/14651858.CD009785.pub2
5. Lally J, MacCabe JH. Antipsychotic medication in schizophrenia: a review. *Br Med Bull.* 2015;114(1):169–179. doi:10.1093/bmb/ldv017
6. Warnez S, Alessi-Severini S. Clozapine: a review of clinical practice guidelines and prescribing trends. *BMC Psychiatry.* 2014;14:102. doi:10.1186/1471-244X-14-102

SOMATIC SYMPTOM AND RELATED DISORDERS

CONVERSION DISORDER (FUNCTIONAL NEUROLOGICAL SYMPTOM DISORDER)

Etiology

The etiology is unknown. Biological factors such as cortisol dysfunction or impaired brain hemisphere communication may be present and continue to be researched.[2] Anxiety and stress also play a role.[1,2] Psychoanalytic theory posits unconscious conflict and the conversion of anxiety into physical symptoms.[2] Childhood abuse or neglect may serve as risk factors.[1] Higher prevalence is seen in rural settings, in those with lower education levels and low socioeconomic status, and in military personnel with combat exposure.[2] A comorbid neurological disease that causes similar symptoms also places individuals at risk.[1,2]

Epidemiology

Prevalence data are unknown but several studies have reported that up to 15% of psychiatric consultations in a general hospital setting are due to conversion disorder.[1,2,6] The onset can occur throughout the life span but is most common between late childhood to early adulthood.[1,2] Conversion disorder is 2 to 3 times more common in females.[1,2]

Clinical Presentation

Individuals typically present with an acute onset of one or more motor or sensory dysfunctions that are often associated with significant stress or trauma. Examples of symptoms include paralysis, blindness, aphonia (mutism), tremor, swallowing or speech symptoms, seizures, weakness, or loss of sensation. The findings suggest a medical condition, but after careful physical examination and diagnostic evaluation, either nothing is found or the findings are not compatible between the symptoms and a medical condition.[1] Neurological disorders frequently co-occur as do depression, anxiety, histrionic personality disorder, and other somatic disorders.[2]

CLINICAL PEARL: The symptoms are not intentionally feigned, as in factitious disorder (to assume the sick role) or malingering (for other secondary gains).[1]

Diagnostic Criteria

- Symptoms of voluntary motor or sensory dysfunction
- The subjective complaint and objective findings are incongruent[1]

Management

- The symptom or deficit often resolves spontaneously, but psychotherapy is useful.[2,6]

- Do not suggest that the symptoms are imaginary or "in their head." Support and education regarding the relationship between stress and physical symptoms are beneficial.[2]

ILLNESS ANXIETY DISORDER

Etiology

The etiology is unknown. Illness anxiety disorder may be precipitated by a significant life stressor or a serious threat to the individual's health that was then determined to be benign.[1,2] A history of childhood abuse or of a serious childhood illness may also serve as risk factors.[1]

Epidemiology

Illness anxiety disorder is formerly known as *hypochondriasis*. The prevalence is similar between males and females. Prevalence estimates are approximately 4% to 6%, but vary and are based upon previous diagnostic terminology of hypochondriasis.[1,2] The onset of symptoms is usually in early or middle adulthood.[1]

Clinical Presentation

Patients are preoccupied with having or acquiring a serious, undiagnosed illness. Unlike somatic symptom disorder, individuals with illness anxiety disorder do not experience a somatic symptom (or do so mildly), but rather they fear that something more severe is going on. They will not be reassured by negative diagnostic testing. They may frequently examine themselves, research the suspected condition, and have high levels of medical utilization.[1] To the opposite extreme, they may avoid appointments or hospitals for fear that something will be detected. The symptoms will be present for at least 6 months, although the illness they fear can change. Depression and anxiety may co-occur.[1]

Diagnostic Criteria

- Fixation with having or getting a serious illness
- If somatic symptoms are present, they are mild[1]

Management

- Treatment of illness anxiety disorder is similar to somatic symptom disorder. Various forms of psychotherapy may be helpful.[2,4]

- Diagnostic tests or procedures should not be ordered unless an underlying medical illness is suspected. Some patients may benefit from frequent and regular appointments for reassurance, whereas others may not.[2]

- Pharmacotherapy for the underlying anxiety may be considered.[2]

SOMATIC SYMPTOM DISORDER

Etiology

The etiology is unknown. Neurotic traits may predispose individuals to developing somatic symptom disorder. Environmental stressors, low socioeconomic status, and lower levels of education are associated with higher rates of the disorder.[1]

Epidemiology

The prevalence in the general population may be approximately 5% to 7% and is higher in females.[1,2] The presence of one prominent symptom is more common in children than adults. The onset of symptoms most commonly occurs in early adulthood. Depression, anxiety, and histrionic personality disorder all co-occur with Somatic symptom disorder.[1,2]

Clinical Presentation

Individuals with somatic symptom disorder experience at least one somatic complaint, such as pain or fatigue, which is disruptive and distressing. Although another medical condition might be present, patients have persistent high levels of worry about illness. Patients may seek care from multiple clinicians and have unusual sensitivities to medications. They may be overly concerned about the significance of the symptoms, or have worry about their health. Finally, they may devote significant time and energy to their symptoms. The disorder will persist for at least 6 months.[1] Depression and increased suicide risk are also associated. In children, the symptoms may consist of abdominal pain, headaches, fatigue, and nausea.[1]

Diagnostic Criteria

- Somatic symptom/s that cause distress to the patient
- Significant worry about the symptoms or their significance[1]

Management

- Note that patients may not seek psychiatric care for somatic symptom disorder, or will resist it if suggested.

- At first, ensure that a medical condition is not the cause of the patient's symptoms. If medical conditions have already been ruled out, further diagnostic evaluations or procedures are discouraged.

- Psychotherapy is recommended. Regular, scheduled appointments are suggested to reassure patients and avoid spontaneous or crisis visits.[2]

- If underlying depression or anxiety is present, pharmacotherapy including SSRIs or SNRIs would be appropriate[2-5]

REFERENCES

1. American Psychiatric Association. *Diagnostic and Statistical Manual of Mental Disorders.* 5th ed. Arlington, VA: American Psychiatric Publishing; 2013.
2. Sadock BJ, Sadock VA, Ruiz P. *Kaplan and Sadock's Synopsis of Psychiatry.* 11th ed. Philadelphia, PA: Wolters Kluwer; 2015.
3. van Dessel N, den Boeft M, van der Wouden JC, et al. Non-pharmacological interventions for somatoform disorders and medically unexplained physical symptoms (MUPS) in adults. *Cochrane Database Syst Rev.* 2014;(11):CD011142. doi:10.1002/14651858.CD011142.pub2
4. Starcevic V. Hypochondriasis: treatment options for a diagnostic quagmire. *Australasian Psychiatry.* 2015;23(4):369–373. doi:10.1177/10398562 15587234

5. Somashekar B, Jainer A, Wuntakal B. Psychopharmacotherapy of somatic symptoms disorders. *Int Rev Psychiatry*. 2013;25(1):107–115. doi:10.3109/09540261.2012.729758
6. Feinstein A. Conversion disorder: advances in our understanding. *Can Med Assoc J*. 2011;183(8):915–920. doi:10.1503/cmaj.110490

SUBSTANCE USE DISORDERS

Etiology

The etiology of substance use disorders is complex; some factors are still being studied.[1,2] Environmental influences, such as availability and social acceptability of a drug, along with peer pressure contribute to the development of a substance use disorder. Personality traits, psychological factors, and family history also influence use. Biological changes in brain structure and neurochemistry are noted but their role is unclear at this time.[2] Dopamine and its role in the reward pathway, as well as the endogenous opioid system and GABA are thought to play a role.[2]

Epidemiology

Cannabis is the most commonly used illicit substance.[3] Other common substances of abuse are alcohol, tobacco, and opioids.[2,3] Comorbidity with other psychiatric disorders, such as depression, is high.[2,3] Specifically, antisocial personality disorder has a high comorbidity with substance use, ranging from 35% to 60% in some studies.[2] In addition, substance abuse has also been found to be a precipitating factor in suicide.[2] Males have higher rates of substance use disorders than females.[1,2] Individuals aged 18 to 24 generally have higher rates of substance use disorders as compared to other age groups.[1]

Clinical Presentation

Substances of abuse produce an intense activation of the reward system (a "high") that results in a pathological pattern of symptoms after continued use.[1] Cognitive, behavioral, and physiological symptoms occur and include impaired control, social impairment, risky use, and tolerance and withdrawal. Individuals may try to decrease or regulate use, but find that they are unsuccessful. Sometimes, all of the day's activities involve the substance. The individual may also withdraw from family or hobbies in order to use, or suffer consequences in school or at their job. Use may occur in potentially hazardous situations such as driving while intoxicated. Despite consequences, the individual fails to abstain from use.[1] Craving also occurs, which is defined as an intense desire or urge for the drug.[1]

Diagnostic Criteria

- Inability to control the use
- Use in risky or hazardous conditions
- Social impairment
- Pharmacological criteria
  - *Tolerance* is the requirement of a higher dose to achieve the same effect, or a reduced effect with the regular dose.[1]
  - Withdrawal occurs after decline or cessation of extended heavy use. Not all substances elicit withdrawal.[1]
- Screening tools
  - The Alcohol Use Disorders Identification Test (AUDIT) and CAGE (cut down/annoyed/guilty/eye opener) questionnaires can be used in screening for alcohol use disorder.

> **CLINICAL PEARL:** Withdrawal symptoms are often the opposite of intoxication symptoms.

Management

- Prevention is the best cure, but specific treatments will be discussed within the sections that follow.
- Overall options include outpatient or inpatient settings where focus is placed on detoxification and/or relapse prevention.
- Self-help groups such as Alcoholics Anonymous (AA) or Narcotics Anonymous (NA) can provide beneficial treatment and support to patients as well.[2]

- Various psychotherapy techniques can be used, and some pharmacological options exist.[2]

- Patients may not be willing to accept treatment at the time you are evaluating them. Multiple factors are involved in a patient's readiness for abstinence. Five stages of behavior change have been described, to include precontemplation, contemplation, preparation, action, and maintenance.[2] Patients may be at various stages of change when you encounter them, and can regress to a previous stage as well.

ALCOHOL AND CENTRAL NERVOUS SYSTEM DEPRESSANTS

This category of substances includes

- Alcohol
- Benzodiazepines and benzodiazepine-like drugs
- Barbiturates
- Hypnotics[1]

The 12-month prevalence for alcohol use disorder in the United States is highest among 18- to 29-year olds. Higher rates are also seen in males, Native Americans/Alaskan Natives, and in those with antisocial personality disorder, bipolar disorder, and schizophrenia.[1] Violence, suicide, and risk of accidents are much higher with alcohol use disorder.[1]

Benzodiazepines are commonly used as anxiolytics. They may also be used to "come down" from a stimulant high, or to increase the high when combined with opioids.[1] Benzodiazepine-like drugs (also referred to as *nonbenzodiazepines*, or *Z-drugs*) such as zolpidem, zaleplon, or eszopiclone are commonly used for insomnia.

> **CLINICAL PEARL:** The central nervous system (CNS) depressants should be used with caution in the elderly population or in those with cognitive impairment. The risk of further confusion or falls is increased.[1]

Intoxication Signs/Symptoms

- Ataxia
- Impaired judgment

- Impaired attention or memory (to include amnesia known as *blackouts*)
- Incoordination
- Slurred speech
- Stupor or coma
- Inappropriate sexual or aggressive behavior
- Nystagmus[1,2]

> **CLINICAL PEARL:** Binge drinking is defined as five or more drinks for males, or four or more for females, on the same occasion on at least 1 day in the past 30 days.[3]

In most states, the level of legal intoxication is 0.08%. At levels of 0.1%, motor function is impaired.[2] At a level of 0.3%, confusion and possibly stupor are present. In nontolerant individuals, blood alcohol levels of approximately 0.4% to 0.5% can lead to death through respiratory or cardiac arrest.[2]

It is important to understand what constitutes "one drink," and to educate patients about this as well. One alcoholic drink contains approximately 14 grams of alcohol. "One drink" includes one 12-ounce beer, one 4- to 5-ounce glass of wine, or 1.5 ounces (a "shot") of distilled spirits such as whiskey, rum, vodka, gin, or tequila.[4]

> **CLINICAL PEARL:** The body can generally metabolize one drink per hour.

Alcohol withdrawal will begin in those who have developed tolerance approximately 4 to 12 hours after cessation or reduction in use.[1,2] The most typical sign of alcohol withdrawal is tremor.[2] The timing of CNS depressant withdrawal will depend upon the half-life of the drug.[1]

Withdrawal Signs/Symptoms

- Anxiety
- Diaphoresis
- Hand tremor
- Insomnia

- Nausea or vomiting
- Tachycardia, hypertension
- Transient visual, tactile, or auditory hallucinations or illusions
- Psychomotor agitation
- Severe: Delirium tremens, generalized tonic–clonic seizures[1,2]

Complications of Alcohol Use Disorder

- Cardiovascular
  - Cardiomyopathy, low-grade hypertension, hypertriglyceridemia, hyperlipidemia[1,2]
- Central and peripheral nervous system
  - Cognitive impairment/dementia, peripheral neuropathy[1,2]
- Gastrointestinal
  - Gastritis, stomach or duodenal ulcers, cirrhosis, or pancreatitis[1,2]

> **CLINICAL PEARL:** Elevations of gamma-glutamyltransferase (GGT) may be seen in those with alcohol use disorder.[1]

- Obstetric
  - Women who are pregnant or breastfeeding should not consume alcohol.

> **CLINICAL PEARL:** Fetal alcohol syndrome is the leading cause of intellectual disability in the United States.[2]

- Vitamin deficiencies
  - Thiamine (B1) deficiency can lead to Wernicke encephalopathy. If untreated, it can progress to Wernicke–Korsakoff syndrome, which involves the inability to form new memories and results in significant cognitive impairment.[2]

> **CLINICAL PEARL:** Classic symptoms of Wernicke encephalopathy include confusion, ataxia, and nystagmus or ocular palsies.[1,2]

Management

- Intoxication
  - A benzodiazepine overdose can be treated with flumazenil, a benzodiazepine antagonist.[2] This medication does have a risk of seizures, and caution should be used.
  - Treatment is otherwise supportive, with monitoring of vital signs and level of consciousness.
- Withdrawal
  - Acute withdrawal from alcohol or CNS depressants should be treated with benzodiazepines.[1,2]

> **CLINICAL PEARL:** The most severe form of alcohol withdrawal is delirium tremens (DTs), which can be life-threatening and is a medical emergency[2] (see Chapter 5, Urgent Management).

  - The Clinical Institute Withdrawal Assessment for Alcohol (CIWA) is a common scale used to assess for withdrawal symptoms.[2]
  - Supplemental thiamine and multivitamins are given.[2]
- Maintenance treatment
  - For maintenance treatment of alcohol use disorder, disulfiram, naltrexone, and acamprosate can be used[2]
- Medical comorbidities discussed earlier in the Complications section need to be considered in the overall management of alcohol use disorder as well. Referral to appropriate specialists is appropriate.
- Psychotherapy modalities are also important components in the treatment of alcohol or CNS depressant use disorders[2]

CAFFEINE

Caffeine is the most widely used behaviorally active drug worldwide.[1,2] It is derived from naturally occurring plant seeds, nuts, or leaves. Sources of caffeine include

- Coffee
- Tea

- Soft drinks
- Beverages marketed as "energy drinks"
- Chocolate
- Over-the-counter analgesics (often marketed for headaches)
- Weight-loss products[1,2]

Adults consume approximately 280 mg of caffeine per day, on average.[1,2] One cup of coffee contains roughly 100 to 150 mg of caffeine. Tea has slightly less, and soft drinks contain up to 50 mg.[2] Energy drinks can have up to 250 mg.[2] Peak concentration occurs in about 30 to 60 minutes, and symptoms last for several hours.[2] Although there is no recognition of caffeine use disorder as compared with the other substances in this discussion, there is established criteria for caffeine intoxication and withdrawal.[1]

Intoxication Signs/Symptoms

- Agitation
- Diuresis
- Excitement
- Flushed face
- Insomnia
- Nervousness
- Gastrointestinal disturbance
- At high doses ($\geq$1 g/d)
  - Muscle twitching
  - Rambling speech
  - Tachycardia or arrhythmia
  - Periods of inexhaustibility[1]

Withdrawal Signs/Symptoms

- Headache
- Depressed or irritable mood
- Fatigue
- Nausea and/or vomiting
- Myalgias or stiffness[1]

> **CLINICAL PEARL:** Headache is the hallmark symptom of caffeine withdrawal.[1]

The headache pain usually comes on gradually, and can be diffuse, throbbing, and sensitive to movement. Withdrawal symptoms usually begin within 12 to 24 hours after the last use, and peak after 1 to 2 days. Withdrawal headaches can last for several weeks.[1]

Complications

Caffeine should be avoided or reduced in anxiety disorders, pregnancy, and gastroesophageal reflux disorder.[2]

Management

- Withdrawal
  - ○ Analgesic medications for a withdrawal headache or symptoms of intoxication are used as needed.[2]
- For patients wanting to reduce or eliminate caffeine, a schedule of decreasing amounts can be created.[2] Eliminating approximately 10 mg per day will reduce withdrawal symptoms.[2]

CANNABIS

Cannabis (marijuana) is derived from the *Cannabis sativa* plant. One of its primary cannabinoids, 1-delta-9 tetrahydrocannabinol (THC), is responsible for the psychoactive effects, which are included in the intoxication list that follows.[1,2] The other main component, cannabidiol, lacks the effects of THC and is being studied for potential therapeutic effects. Synthetic forms of THC are approved by the FDA for chemotherapy-induced nausea and vomiting.[1] There has also been interest in using cannabis for other medical conditions; however, it is important to note that it is not currently recommended as first-line therapy for any medical condition. Other synthetic forms are used recreationally and are known as "K2" or "spice."[1] One of the concerns regarding cannabis, be it for recreational or medicinal use, is the variability in potency and the fact that the potency has increased over time.[1] A common myth among laypersons is that cannabis is not addictive; however, dependence does occur.[2]

Cannabis is typically rolled into a cigarette, also referred to as a *joint*, and smoked.[2] Pipes and water pipes (bongs, hookahs) are also used for smoking. Vaporizing, or vaping, has become a recent trend, in which a device heats the substance, which can then be inhaled without the presence of smoke.[5] Cannabis can also be formulated into oils, foods, and beverages.[2]

Regarding toxicology screens, cannabis can be detected in urine, blood, saliva, and hair. Cannabinoids are fat soluble and are excreted slowly. Positive results have been seen up to 30 days after the last use in chronic, heavy users. Note that secondhand smoke exposure will not result in a positive drug screen.[2]

CLINICAL PEARL: Cannabis is the most commonly used illicit substance worldwide.[1,2] Of all the psychoactive drugs, it follows caffeine, alcohol, and nicotine as the fourth most commonly used substance.[2]

Intoxication Signs/Symptoms

- Conjunctival injection
- Dry mouth
- Increased appetite or food cravings
- Impaired motor coordination
- Euphoria
- Tachycardia
- Anxiety or paranoia
- Sensation of slowed time
- Impaired judgment
- Social withdrawal[1]

Withdrawal Signs/Symptoms

- Irritability, anger, or depression
- Anxiety or restlessness
- Insomnia or distressing dreams
- Decreased appetite or weight loss
- Abdominal pain
- Tremors
- Diaphoresis, fever, or chills
- Headache[1]

Complications

- Insomnia from withdrawal may last up to 1 month
- Chronic cough or other respiratory symptoms can occur from smoking cannabis
- An "amotivational syndrome" has been described as a result of use, in which social and goal-directed activities are reduced
- Reproductive effects
- Psychosis can also be induced or exacerbated by cannabis[1,2]

Management

- There are no pharmacologic agents for the treatment of cannabis use disorder. Intoxication and withdrawal are not life-threatening.[2]
- Approximately 10 % of regular marijuana users will become dependent, with adolescents being most susceptible.[2,6]
- Motor impairment occurs with cannabis use; individuals should be educated to avoid driving while intoxicated.[2,6]
- Psychotherapy with counseling and support should be offered.

HALLUCINOGENS

Hallucinogens are composed of natural and synthetic substances. They are also referred to as *psychedelics*.[2] Some examples include

- Lysergic acid diethylamide (LSD, "acid")
- 3, 4- methylenedioxymethamphetamine (MDMA, "ecstasy")
  - ○ MDMA is also considered an amphetamine
- Psilocybin
- Mescaline
- Morning glory seeds
- Jimsonweed
- Salvia divinorum[1]

Although the current incidence of hallucinogen use is not as common as other substances of abuse, hallucinogens can have deleterious effects. High rates of use were seen in the late 1960s with LSD, and in the late 1990s with MDMA.[2] Withdrawal from hallucinogens has been observed in animal studies but has not been defined in humans; therefore, withdrawal criteria are not listed within this category.[1]

Intoxication Signs/Symptoms

- Anxiety or depression
- Ideas of reference
- Illusions or hallucinations
- Depersonalization or derealization
- Fear of "losing one's mind"
- Paranoia
- Mydriasis and/or blurred vision
- Tachycardia or palpitations
- Diaphoresis
- Tremors
- Incoordination
- Impaired judgment[1]

Phencyclidine (PCP, "angel dust") and other similar substances, such as ketamine, are also categorized as hallucinogens. They have a slightly different set of intoxication symptoms. Violent behavior can occur perhaps because patients feel that they are being attacked.[1]

Intoxication Signs/Symptoms

- Violent
- Belligerent
- Impulsive
- Nystagmus
- Hypertension or tachycardia
- Numbness or reduced sensitivity to pain
- Ataxia
- Muscular rigidity
- Seizures or coma
- Hyperacusis[1]

Complications

- Users may experience a "bad trip" while intoxicated, which can consist of anxious and/or psychotic symptoms.[2]

- After using hallucinogens, individuals can experience a "flashback" in the absence of intoxication. This experience is usually brief (seconds to minutes), but may last for weeks or up to years.[1,2] The long-lasting effect is also referred to as a *persistent perceptual disorder*[1]
  - In a flashback, perceptual disturbances (most often visual), are reexperienced while the patient is sober.
  - The perceptions can include hallucinations of shapes or movement in peripheral vision, intensified colors, flashes of color, afterimages, halos, macropsia, or micropsia. This occurs most often following the use of LSD, but can occur with any of the hallucinogens.[1]
- Cognitive deficits
- Cardiovascular risks include cardiac arrest
- Rhabdomyolysis
- Intracranial bleeding
- Respiratory effects
- Neurological disorders[1]

Management

- Intoxication
  - During intoxication, reassurance and supportive care should be provided.[2] Sensory stimulation should be eliminated as much as possible.[2]
  - Benzodiazepines can be administered to help relieve symptoms of an unpleasant intoxication.[2,7]
  - If the patient is violent during intoxication, restraints may be necessary to protect the patient or others, but should be avoided when possible.
  - MDMA also has stimulant effects, which would need to be considered in the evaluation or treatment of intoxication.[2]
- For a persistent perceptual disorder, benzodiazepines and anticonvulsants have been utilized, but symptoms may persist as there is no drug that has been found to be completely efficacious in eliminating symptoms.[2,7]
- Antipsychotics can be used if psychotic symptoms persist after hallucinogen use, but should be avoided during the intoxication phase.[2]

INHALANTS

Inhalants are toxic gases from products such as glues, fuels, and paints or paint thinners that produce a high.[1,2] Other common household products used as inhalants include whipped cream canisters, vegetable oil cooking spray, and nail polish remover. Specific chemicals within the inhalant products can include acetone, butane, fluorocarbons, propane, or toluene.[1] Inhalants are also referred to as "volatile" substances or "solvents."[2] Nitrite inhalants "poppers" and nitrous oxide "laughing gas" are not included in this section but can have similar effects.[2]

The prevalence of use is higher in those aged 12 to 17; the products are often inexpensive and easy to obtain.[1,2,8] Conduct disorder, ADHD, depressive disorders, or PTSD are often comorbid with inhalant use.[2] Standard toxicology screens do not detect inhalants.[1] Inhalants generally act as CNS depressants.[2] Withdrawal symptoms are uncommon and mild, and are not included as criteria in the *DSM-5*.[1]

The use of inhalants typically involves sniffing, huffing, or bagging[1,2]

- Sniffing is the breathing in of a substance directly from the container

- Huffing involves saturating a cloth with the substance and inhaling it while placed over the mouth and the nose

- Bagging is inhaling the fumes of a substance that have been poured or placed into a bag[1]

Intoxication Signs/Symptoms

- Violence

- Nystagmus

- Incoordination, ataxia

- Slurred speech

- Lethargy

- Diminished reflexes

- Psychomotor retardation

- Tremor

- Weakness

- Blurred vision or diplopia

- Stupor or coma
- Euphoria[1]

Complications

- A "sudden sniffing death" has been reported, which is thought to be due to cardiac arrhythmia or arrest[1]
- Renal, hepatic, and neurologic complications can also occur[1]

Management

- Intoxication
  - Treatment of inhalant intoxication is supportive. Respiratory and cardiac function should be monitored[2,8]
  - Benzodiazepines and other sedatives will worsen the intoxication and are contraindicated[2]
- Psychotherapy can be offered, as well as day treatment or residential programs.[2,8] Family therapy should also be offered[8]

NON–SUBSTANCE-RELATED DISORDERS: GAMBLING DISORDER

Although there are other addictive behaviors that occur without the ingestion of substances, at this time there is only evidence to support the inclusion of gambling disorder within this category in the *DSM-5*. Some individuals suffer significant impairment related to gambling, including suicidal ideation. Note that if these behaviors occur in the context of a manic episode, the more appropriate diagnosis is bipolar disorder.[1]

OPIOIDS

Opioids have been utilized throughout history as analgesics, but are commonly misused to obtain a recreational high.[2] Some examples of natural and synthetic opioids include

- Heroin
- Morphine
- Methadone
- Fentanyl

- Codeine
- Oxycodone[1,2]

The number of individuals in the United States with opioid use disorder exceeds two million.[9] Rates of overdose deaths have risen dramatically over the last two decades as well. Opioid use disorder is often comorbid with depression, anxiety, alcohol use disorder, and antisocial personality disorder.[2]

Intoxication Signs/Symptoms

- Miosis
- Drowsiness ("nod") or coma
- Respiratory depression
- Slurred speech
- Constipation
- Nausea
- Impairment in attention or memory
- Initial euphoria, can become dysphoric
- Apathy
- Impaired judgment[1]

> **CLINICAL PEARL:** Common signs of an opioid overdose are respiratory depression, altered mental status/coma, and miosis.[2,10]

Withdrawal Signs/Symptoms

- Nausea, vomiting, or diarrhea
- Myalgias
- Lacrimation or rhinorrhea
- Midriasis
- Piloerection
- Diaphoresis
- Yawning
- Fever

- Depression
- Insomnia[1]

Complications

- Those with opioid use disorder who use intravenously are at risk for cellulitis, hepatitis, HIV infection, and endocarditis[1,2]
- Individuals may resort to subcutaneous injections ("skin popping") when veins become sclerosed and unavailable[2]
- Death from overdose is common, usually from respiratory arrest[2]

Management

- Overdose
  - Naloxone, an opioid antagonist, is administered in an opioid overdose.[2,10] It works quickly and effectively to bind to the opioid receptors
- Withdrawal
  - Acute withdrawal is rarely fatal and is treated symptomatically. Clonidine can be used for hypertension, and other agents as needed for symptomatic relief of abdominal cramps and/or diarrhea[2]
  - A common objective scale to assess opioid withdrawal is the Clinical Opioid Withdrawal Scale (COWS)
- Maintenance treatment
  - Medication-assisted treatment (MAT) is an approach to treating substances use disorders that combines pharmacotherapy and psychotherapy. MAT can only be dispensed at approved opioid treatment programs (OTP)[11]
  - Methadone or buprenorphine are commonly utilized as MAT in the maintenance treatment of opioid use disorder[2,9]
    - Methadone is a synthetic opioid and is administered orally in approved clinics. It suppresses withdrawal symptoms and allows the individual to detoxify more easily over a period of time, without the risk of continued illicit intravenous use[2]
      - Note that methadone has to be separately assessed on toxicology screens, and will not cause a positive result within general opioid toxicology screens

- Buprenorphine is an oral opioid agonist medication that is approved for opioid use disorder.[2,9] It weakens or blocks the effects of opioids. It can be combined with naloxone to decrease the potential for misuse

  - Buprenorphine can be prescribed following the completion of an approved training program and application of a waiver from the drug enforcement agency (DEA)[2,11]

  - Naltrexone is an opioid antagonist, similar to naloxone, which decreases cravings in opioid and alcohol use disorders. Naltrexone is not used in opioid overdoses because it does not bind as quickly to the receptors as naloxone does[11]

- Psychotherapy techniques, including individual behavioral, family, and support groups, are also recommended for opioid use disorder[2,11]

Stimulants

The stimulant category of substances encompasses cocaine, amphetamines, and other drugs such as MDMA, which is also considered a hallucinogen as discussed earlier.[1,2] Cocaine is used medically for its anesthetic and vasoconstrictive properties.[2] An interesting fact is that cocaine was also used as the active ingredient in Coca-Cola until the early 1900s.[2] It has significant addictive qualities, and users can develop psychological dependence after only one use.[2] Crack is cocaine that has been converted into its base form, and is also highly addictive.[2]

Prescription amphetamines can be utilized in the treatment of ADHD, obesity, and narcolepsy.[1,2] Amphetamines, however, are commonly abused illicit substances.[2] Examples of amphetamine and amphetamine-like substances include

- Dextroamphetamine
- Methamphetamine
- Methylphenidate
- Pseudoephedrine
- Modafinil[1,2]

Over-the-counter availability of pseudoephedrine is now regulated, as it was being used to make methamphetamine.[2] In general, these substances should be used with caution in patients with hypertension, as they can raise blood pressure.[2] Some stimulants can also precipitate psychosis, often with paranoia, ideas of reference, or auditory or tactile hallucinations.[2]

Intoxication Signs/Symptoms

- Euphoria
- Hypervigilance
- Midriasis
- Impaired judgment
- Diaphoresis or chills
- Nausea or vomiting
- Weight loss
- Anxiety or aggression
- Respiratory depression
- Chest pain or cardiac arrhythmias
- Hyperpyrexia
- Confusion, seizures, dyskinesias, dystonias, or coma
- At higher doses: headache or tinnitus[1]

Withdrawal Signs/Symptoms:

- Fatigue
- Increased appetite
- Depression or suicidal ideation
- Bad dreams
- Sleep disturbances[1]

Complications

- Myocardial infarction, arrhythmias, and cardiac arrest
- Respiratory illnesses, infections, or arrest
- Weight loss
- Malnutrition
- Intranasal use can lead to sinusitis, irritation or bleeding of the mucosa, or a perforated nasal septum
- Psychosis

- Higher risk of HIV infection, hepatitis, and tuberculosis[1,2]
- Methamphetamine use, specifically, can cause cognitive impairment as well as tooth decay and oral lesions known as "meth mouth"[1,12]

Management

- There are no specific pharmacologic agents for the intoxication or withdrawal of stimulant use disorder[2,13]
- Antipsychotics or benzodiazepines may be used symptomatically.[2]
- Psychotherapy methods including individual, group, and family are recommended[2,13]

TOBACCO

Tobacco use contributes to significant mortality rates and healthcare costs.[2] Cigarettes are the most common form of tobacco used by individuals.[1,2] Approximately 20% of individuals in the United States smoke.[2] Other tobacco products include cigars, smokeless (chewing) tobacco, and pipes.[1,2] Symptoms of tobacco use disorder include smoking shortly after waking, increasing the amount of cigarettes smoked per day, and waking at night to smoke.[1]

The primary psychoactive substance in tobacco is nicotine.[2] Nicotine can be measured in blood, saliva, or urine.[1] Other substance use disorders, mood disorders, and personality disorders are often comorbid with tobacco use disorder.[1] There are no diagnostic criteria for intoxication, but withdrawal from nicotine results in common symptoms as noted here.[1]

Withdrawal Signs/Symptoms

- Anxiety or depression
- Irritability
- Increased appetite
- Insomnia
- Difficulty concentrating[1]

Complications

Cardiovascular illnesses, chronic obstructive pulmonary disease (COPD), and cancers are the most common complications of smoking/tobacco use.[1] Pregnant women who smoke are at risk for low-birth-weight newborns.[1]

Management

- Most individuals have tried to quit on at least one occasion[2]
- A "quit date" can be recommended, but if patients prefer gradual cessation, this should be respected[2]
- Nicotine replacement using over-the-counter patches, gum, or lozenges are useful[2,14]
- Non-nicotine prescription medications such as bupropion and varenicline can be used as well[2,14]
- Behavioral and/or group therapy can be successful and are recommended in conjunction with pharmacotherapy[2,14]

REFERENCES

1. American Psychiatric Association. *Diagnostic and Statistical Manual of Mental Disorders.* 5th ed. Arlington, VA: American Psychiatric Publishing; 2013.
2. Sadock BJ, Sadock VA, Ruiz P. *Kaplan and Sadock's Synopsis of Psychiatry.* 11th ed. Philadelphia, PA: Wolters Kluwer; 2015.
3. Substance Abuse and Mental Health Services Administration. Key substance use and mental health indicators in the United States: results from the 2016 national survey on drug use and health. https://www.samhsa .gov/data/report/key-substance-use-and-mental-health-indicators -united-states-results-2016-national-survey
4. National Institutes of Health. What is a standard drink? https://www .niaaa.nih.gov/alcohol-health/overview-alcohol-consumption/what -standard-drink
5. Owen K, Sutter M, Albertson T. Marijuana: respiratory tract effects. *Clin Rev Allergy Immunol.* 2014;46(1):65–81. doi:10.1007/s12016-013-8374-y
6. Volkow N, Baler R, Compton W, Weiss S. Adverse health effects of marijuana use. *N Engl J Med.* 2014;370(23):2219–2227. doi:10.1056/ NEJMra1402309
7. Lerner AG, Gelkopf M, Skladman I, et al. Flashback and hallucinogen persisting perception disorder: clinical aspects and pharmacological treatment approach. *Isr J Psychiatry Relat Sci.* 2002;39(2):92–99.
8. Ford JB, Sutter ME, Owen KP, Albertson TE. Volatile substance misuse: an updated review of toxicity and treatment. *Clin Rev Allergy Immunol.* 2014;46(1):19–33. doi:10.1007/s12016-013-8371-1
9. Thomas CP, Fullerton CA, Kim M, et al. Medication-assisted treatment with buprenorphine: assessing the evidence. *Psychiatr Serv.* 2014;65(2):158–170. doi:10.1176/appi.ps.201300256

10. Boyer EW. Management of opioid analgesic overdose. *N Engl J Med.* 2012;367(2):146–155. doi:10.1056/NEJMra1202561

11. Substance Abuse and Mental Health Services Administration. Medication and counseling treatment. https://www.samhsa.gov/medication -assisted-treatment/treatment. Updated May 7, 2019.

12. Shetty VS, Mooney LJ, Zigler CM, et al. The relationship between methamphetamine use and increased dental disease. *J Am Dent Assoc.* 2010;141(3):307–318. doi:10.14219/jada.archive.2010.0165

13. Minozzi S, Saulle R, De Crescenzo F, Amato L. Psychosocial interventions for psychostimulant misuse. *Cochrane Database Syst Rev.* 2016;(9):CD011866. doi:10.1002/14651858.CD011866.pub2

14. Stead LF, Koilpillai P, Fanshawe TR, Lancaster T. Combined pharmacotherapy and behavioural interventions for smoking cessation. *Cochrane Database Syst Rev.* 2016;(3):CD008286. doi:10.1002/14651858 .CD008286.pub3

TRAUMA AND STRESSOR-RELATED DISORDERS

ADJUSTMENT DISORDER

Etiology

Adjustment disorders are precipitated by a stressor. Responses to stressors vary and are affected by the individual's personality characteristics, cultural norms, and genetic and familial factors.[1]

Epidemiology

Adjustment disorders occur commonly in both outpatient and inpatient settings. The prevalence in the general population ranges from 2% to 8%.[1] The disorders are diagnosed most commonly in adolescents. Increased prevalence is seen in women.[1,2] In adults, common stressors include marital conflict, relocating, or finances. In adolescents, school issues, parental divorce, and substance use are common stressors.[1]

Clinical Presentation

Adjustment disorders are defined by the development of emotional or behavioral symptoms following an identifiable stressor. The reaction is out of proportion to the stressor and may contain depressive, anxiety, and/or behavioral symptoms.[1,2] Physical symptoms, reckless behaviors, or suicidal ideation can also occur.[1] The symptoms are not a component of normal bereavement and do not persist for more than 6 months once the stressor has ended.[2]

Diagnostic Criteria

- Distress that is out of proportion to the stressor
- The symptoms do not meet the criteria for another mental disorder[2]
  - For example, if the patient meets criteria for the diagnosis of MDD in the context of a stressor, then MDD would be the more appropriate diagnosis

Management

- Psychotherapy is the treatment of choice for adjustment disorders.[1,3] Group or individual therapy has been found to be beneficial[1]
- The efficacy of pharmacotherapy has not been studied, but anxiolytics or antidepressants are presumed to be appropriate for a limited time if needed[1,3]

POSTTRAUMATIC STRESS DISORDER

Etiology

The etiology of PTSD is unknown. Potential biological factors include dysfunction in the noradrenergic or opioid system, or the hypothalamic pituitary adrenal (HPA) axis.[1] Risk factors include prior psychiatric history, lower socioeconomic status, low education levels, exposure to previous trauma, and female sex.[2]

Epidemiology

The lifetime prevalence of PTSD in the general population is approximately 8%.[1] Twelve-month prevalence is approximately 3.5% in U.S. adults.[2] Higher rates are seen in veterans, first responders, and survivors of rape, internment, or genocide.[2]

Clinical Presentation

PTSD is characterized by the development of variable symptom categories following exposure to one or more traumatic events. Patients will experience intrusion symptoms including dreams or flashbacks and will avoid reminders of the trauma. They will experience dysphoric mood states or amnesia for the event. Irritability, increased startle response, and difficulty concentrating can also be seen. Note that symptoms differ in children. Suicidal ideation or attempts may occur. Common comorbidities include mood and other anxiety disorders, as well as substance use disorders.[1,2] To differentiate from acute stress disorder, the duration of the disturbance is more than 1 month.[2]

> **CLINICAL PEARL:** A similar diagnosis, acute stress disorder, consists of comparable symptoms but occurs from 3 days to 1 month following the trauma.[2]

Diagnostic Criteria

- Exposure to death, serious injury, or sexual violence
- Avoidance of stimuli associated with the trauma
- Intrusion symptoms such as memories, nightmares, or flashbacks
- Symptoms of hyperarousal, such as hypervigilance or exaggerated startle response
- Negative thoughts or mood, such as feeling guilty or blaming self[2]

Management

- There are no current recommended treatments to prevent PTSD following a trauma[4]
- The recommended first-line treatment for PTSD is SSRIs.[1,5] Two tricyclic antidepressants, imipramine and amitriptyline, have also demonstrated efficacy[1]
- Prazosin, an alpha-blocker, has been used for nightmares

- Various psychotherapies may be effective for patients as well. Research is ongoing, but trauma-focused CBT and eye movement desensitization and reprocessing have been used[4]

REFERENCES

1. Sadock BJ, Sadock VA, Ruiz P. *Kaplan and Sadock's Synopsis of Psychiatry.* 11th ed. Philadelphia, PA: Wolters Kluwer; 2015.
2. American Psychiatric Association. *Diagnostic and Statistical Manual of Mental Disorders.* 5th ed. Arlington, VA: American Psychiatric Publishing; 2013.
3. Carta MG, Balestrieri M, Murru A, Hardoy MC. Adjustment disorder: epidemiology, diagnosis and treatment. *Clin Practice Epidemiol Ment Health.* 2009;5:15. doi:10.1186/1745-0179-5-15
4. Bisson JI, Cosgrove S, Lewis C, Roberts NP. Post-traumatic stress disorder. *BMJ.* 2015;351:h6161. doi:10.1136/bmj.h6161
5. Stein DJ, Ipser JC, Seedat S, et al. Pharmacotherapy for post traumatic stress disorder (PTSD). *Cochrane Database Syst Rev.* 2006;(1):CD002795. doi:10.1002/14651858.CD002795.pub2

ELECTRONIC RESOURCES

The World Professional Association for Transgender Health Standards of Care.

https://www.wpath.org/publications/soc

Endocrine Society Clinical Practice Guideline for Endocrine Treatment of Gender-Dysphoric/Gender-Incongruent Persons.

https://www.endocrine.org/guidelines-and-clinical-practice/clinical -practice-guidelines/gender-dysphoria-gender-incongruence

3

Diagnostic Testing

Introduction

Although there are no confirmatory diagnostic studies for any of the psychiatric illnesses, diagnostic tests may still be warranted. It is important to order diagnostic studies to rule out medical conditions that may present with psychiatric symptoms or to evaluate somatic symptom disorders. In addition, labs, imaging, or procedures can establish normal levels or baseline functioning, which is important when considering pharmacotherapy or other treatment decisions.

Despite the lack of diagnostic tests to confirm psychiatric disorders, a number of psychiatric rating scales exist that can assist with diagnosis. Some are more appropriate for research as opposed to practical clinical settings, but several common scales are described.

Patients who present for psychiatric treatment often require medical assessments to rule out physical causes for their symptoms. The medical tests listed in Table 3.1 are those commonly requested.

TABLE 3.1 Common Laboratory Evaluations

Name	Normal Reference Range	Indication	Interpretation
B12 level	200–600 pg/mL	Screening	B12 may be deficient in alcohol use disorder
Blood alcohol level	≤0	Screening	Levels between 0.30 and 0.40 g/dL can be fatal

(continued)

TABLE 3.1 Common Laboratory Evaluations (*continued*)

Name	Normal Reference Range	Indication	Interpretation
BUN and creatinine	BUN: 7–18 mg/dL Creatinine: 0.6–1.2 mg/dL	Screening or for lithium clearance	Renal impairment may reduce lithium clearance
Complete blood count	WBC: 4,500–11,000/mm^3	Screening or for clozapine	Clozapine carries risk of agranulocytosis
Electrolytes	Sodium: 136–145 mEq/L Chloride: 95–105 mEq/L Potassium: 3.5–5.0 mEq/L Bicarbonate: 22–28 mEq/L Magnesium: 1.5–2.0 mEq/L	Eating disorders or alcohol use disorder	May be abnormal in eating disorders or alcohol use disorder
Folate level	3–20 ng/mL	Screening	May be reduced in alcohol use disorders
GGT	0–30 IU/L	Screening for alcohol use disorder	May be elevated in heavy drinkers
Hepatitis panel	Varied components	Screening	Infection with hepatitis may affect psychiatric symptoms and impact treatment
Liver function tests	Alanine aminotransferase (ALT, GPT, SGPT): 8–20 U/L Alkaline phosphatase: 20–70 U/L Aspartate aminotransferase (AST, GOT, SGOT): 8–20 U/L	Screening	Hepatic impairment will affect choice of pharmacological agents
Medication levels (acetaminophen, salicylate, mood stabilizers, antidepressants)	Varied components	Monitor toxicity or compliance	Evaluate levels to assess for overdose, toxicity, and/or compliance

(*continued*)

TABLE 3.1 Common Laboratory Evaluations (*continued*)

Name	Normal Reference Range	Indication	Interpretation
Prolactin level	<20 ng/mL	Following a seizure or to monitor as a side effect of antipsychotic medications	Antipsychotic medications may cause hyperprolactinemia
RPR	Positive or negative	Syphilis screen	If positive, follow up with confirmatory testing using FTA-ABS or TP-PA
Thyroid function tests	Thyroid-stimulating hormone: 0.5–5.0 μU/mL Thyroxine (T4): 5–12 mcg/dL Triiodothyronine (T3): 115–190 ng/dL	Screening	Abnormalities in thyroid function can contribute to psychiatric symptoms
Toxicology screens— most commonly from urine sample	Positive or negative	For unexplained behavioral symptoms, monitoring abstinence, or as a general screen	Interpretations indicate presence or absence of substances
Urinalysis	Varied components	Screening	Urinary tract infections can contribute to confusion or delirium in the elderly

ALT, alanine aminotransferase; AST, aspartate aminotransferase; BUN, blood urea nitrogen; FTA-ABS, fluorescent treponemal antibody absorption test; GGT, gamma-glutamyltransferase; GOT, glutamic-oxalocetic transaminase; GPT, glutamic pyruvic transaminase; RPR, rapid plasma reagin; SGOT, serum glutamic oxaloacetic transaminase; SGPT, serum glutamic pyruvic transaminase; TP-PA, T pallidum particle agglutination; WBC, white blood cell.

DIAGNOSTIC IMAGING STUDIES

COMPUTED TOMOGRAPHY (CT)

Head

- Indication: To rule out medical comorbidities, such as stroke, subdural hematoma, tumor, or abscess, that may cause psychiatric symptoms.

MAGNETIC RESONANCE IMAGING (MRI)

Head

- Indication: To rule out medical comorbidities, such as vascular malformations, infarctions, or neoplasms, that may cause psychiatric symptoms.

OTHER DIAGNOSTIC TESTING

ELECTROCARDIOGRAM (ECG)

- Indication: For screening of underlying cardiac abnormalities or electroconvulsive therapy (ECT) clearance.

ELECTROENCEPHALOGRAM (EEG)

- Indication: To rule out a seizure disorder.

Psychiatric Rating Scales and Screening Tools

A variety of rating scales or screening tools exist as questionnaires, interviews, or checklists[1]; some are clinician-administered, whereas others can be self-administered; those commonly used are listed as follows.

Alcohol Use Disorder

Alcohol Use Disorders Identification Test (AUDIT)

- This 10-item questionnaire screens for harmful alcohol consumption. It was developed by the World Health Organization and is appropriate for primary care settings.[2]

CAGE Questionnaire

- Four questions serve as a brief screen. Each "yes" answer is 1 point. A score of 1 warrants follow-up; a score of ≥2 strongly suggests a problem.[1,2]
  - Have you ever felt you should **C**ut down on your drinking?
  - Have people **A**nnoyed you by criticizing your drinking?
  - Have you ever felt **G**uilty about your drinking?
  - Have you ever had a drink first thing in the morning to steady your nerves or to get rid of a hangover? (**E**ye-opener)

Anxiety

Hamilton Anxiety Rating Scale (HAM-A)

- This scale assesses overall somatic and cognitive anxiety symptoms.[1]

Panic Disorder Severity Scale (PDSS)

- This seven-item scale specifically addresses symptoms of panic attacks.[1]

Yale–Brown Obsessive-Compulsive Scale (YBOCS)

- This 10-item assessment for obsessive-compulsive disorder (OCD) symptoms is standard in research and can be used clinically to gage treatment response.[1]

ATTENTION DEFICIT HYPERACTIVITY DISORDER

Conners Rating Scales

- These scales are used in screening for attention deficit hyperactivity disorder (ADHD) and are available in parent and teacher versions as well as a self-report for adolescents.[1]

Vanderbilt Assessment Scales

- These parent and teacher scales assess for symptoms of ADHD and other comorbid conditions such as oppositional defiant disorder, conduct disorder, and anxiety/depression.

AUTISM

Autism Diagnostic Interview-Revised (ADI-R)

- This scale is used widely in research and may have use in a clinical setting.[1]

Modified Checklist for Autism in Toddlers, Revised With Follow-Up (M-CHAT-R/F)

- This screening tool is validated for children between 16 and 30 months of age.

BIPOLAR DISORDER

Mood Disorder Questionnaire

- This screening tool includes 13 questions regarding symptoms of bipolar disorder.[2]

COGNITIVE DISORDERS

Mini-Mental Status Examination (MMSE)

- This 30-point test assesses cognition and was widely used and distributed until it was copyrighted in 2001.[1] Different versions of the test are now utilized more frequently, including the Montreal Cognitive Assessment (MoCA).

DEPRESSION

Beck Depression Inventory (BDI)

- This self-report scale is used in clinical trials and sometimes as a screening tool for major depression.[1]

Hamilton Rating Scale for Depression (HAM-D)

- This objective scale is commonly used in research and to evaluate symptom response to treatment.[1]

Patient Health Questionnaire-9 (PHQ-9)

- This subjective scale can assist in screening or facilitating diagnosis.[1]

Zung Self-Rating Depression Scale

- This 20-item subjective scale can assist in the identification of depressive symptoms.[1]

EATING DISORDERS

Bulimia Test-Revised (BULIT-R)

- This assessment is useful in screening for bulimia nervosa.[1]

Eating Disorders Examination (EDE-Q)

- This is a self-report version of a longer scale, which has use if an eating disorder is suspected.[1]

INTELLECTUAL TESTING

Wechsler Intelligence Scales/Stanford-Binet Intelligence Scale (SB)

- The intelligence quotient (IQ) can be measured with either of these tests. Intelligence tests evaluate factors such as comprehension, math skills, vocabulary, and others.[1]

PERSONALITY DISORDERS

Personality Disorder Questionnaire (PDQ)

- This self-report questionnaire includes 85 yes/no questions to assess for personality disorders.[1]

PROJECTIVE PERSONALITY TESTS

Rorschach

- This well-known assessment contains 10 cards of symmetrical inkblots that are interpreted by patients. It is utilized to assess for thought disorders or defense mechanisms.[1]

Thematic Apperception Test (TAT)

- The patient is asked to create a story based upon images of individuals in various situations. This can provide insight into the motivations behind patient behaviors.[1]

PSYCHOSIS

Positive and Negative Syndrome Scale (PANSS)

- The Positive and Negative Syndrome Scale (PANSS) is a standard scale for clinical outcomes in research and is also helpful in assessing the severity of symptoms in clinical practice.[1]

Tardive Dyskinesia

The Abnormal Involuntary Movement Scale (AIMS)

- The Abnormal Involuntary Movement Scale (AIMS) is a clinician-administered and scored assessment for tardive dyskinesia in patients being treated with antipsychotic medications. Evaluation of facial and oral extremity and trunk movements as well as a global judgment and dental status is completed.[1]

References

1. Sadock BJ, Sadock VA, Ruiz P. *Kaplan and Sadock's Synopsis of Psychiatry.* 11th ed. Philadelphia, PA: Wolters Kluwer; 2015.
2. SAMHSA HRSA Center for Integrated Health Solutions. Screening Tools. https://www.integration.samhsa.gov/clinical-practice/screening-tools

Electronic Resources

AIMS evaluation

> http://www.cqaimh.org/pdf/tool_aims.pdf

Alcohol Use Disorders Identification Test (AUDIT)

> https://www.integration.samhsa.gov/AUDIT_screener_for_alcohol.pdf

Beck Depression Inventory (BDI)

> https://www.ismanet.org/doctoryourspirit/pdfs/Beck-Depression-Inventory-BDI.pdf

Cage Questionnaire

> https://www.integration.samhsa.gov/images/res/CAGEAID.pdf

Eating Disorders Examination (EDE-Q)

> http://cedd.org.au/wordpress/wp-content/uploads/2014/09/Eating-Disorder-Examination-Questionnaire-EDE-Q.pdf

Hamilton Anxiety Rating Scale (HAM-A)

> https://dcf.psychiatry.ufl.edu/files/2011/05/HAMILTON-ANXIETY.pdf, http://www.assessmentpsychology.com/HAM-A.pdf

Hamilton Rating Scale for Depression (HAM-D)

> https://www.outcometracker.org/library/HAM-D.pdf

Modified Checklist for Autism in Toddlers, Revised with Follow-Up (M-CHAT-R/F)

>https://cms.m-chat.org/LineagenMChat/media/Lineagen-M-Chat-Media/mchatDOTorg.pdf

Montreal Cognitive Assessment (MoCA)

>http://dhhs.ne.gov/children_family_services/ProtectionSafety Policy/APS%20Policy/MoCA-Test-English%207.1.pdf

Mood Disorders Questionnaire (MDQ)2

>https://www.integration.samhsa.gov/images/res/MDQ.pdf

Panic Disorder Severity Scale (PDSS)

>http://www.goodmedicine.org.uk/files/panic,%20assessment%20pdss.pdf

Patient Health Questionnaire-9 (PHQ-9)

>https://www.integration.samhsa.gov/images/res/PHQ%20-%20Questions.pdf

Personality Disorder Questionnaire (PDQ)

>http://www.pdq4.com

Positive and Negative Syndrome Scale (PANSS)

>http://medavante.vo.llnwd.net/v1/External/MedAvante/PANSS/English/RPE/MedAvante_PANSS_SCI-PANSS_1999_English.pdf

Stanford–Binet Intelligence Scale (SB)

>https://stanfordbinettest.com

Vanderbilt Assessment Scales

>https://www.nichq.org/sites/default/files/resource-file/NICHQ-Vanderbilt-Assessment-Scales.pdf

Wechsler Intelligence Scales

>https://wechsleriqtest.com

Yale–Brown Obsessive-Compulsive Scale (YBOCS)

>http://tacanow.org/wp-content/uploads/2013/05/YBOC-Symptom-Checklist.pdf

Zung Self-Rating Depression Scale

>http://www.mentalhealthministries.net/resources/flyers/zung_scale/zung_scale.pdf

4

Patient Education and Counseling

Introduction

Patient education topics in individuals with psychiatric illnesses are as important as in other medical settings. Health-maintenance and disease-prevention topics can be discussed with patients, as appropriate and indicated. Proper diet, exercise, and sleep patterns are essential to not only physical health but mental health as well. In addition, patients with serious mental illnesses tend to have poorer physical health than the general population. Following is a discussion of areas that are specific to psychiatry.

SELECTED PATIENT EDUCATION TOPICS PERTINENT TO PSYCHIATRY

DEFENSE MECHANISMS

Defense mechanisms can be used by all persons (with or without psychiatric illness) as a means to cope, protect, and/or reduce anxiety about conflicts. Freud viewed defense mechanisms as generally unconscious processes utilized by the ego. Freudian theory describes the ego as the mediator between the id and the superego; the id being primitive and pleasure-seeking unconscious thoughts, and the superego being the conscience and the ideal morality.[1]

Defense mechanisms can be categorized as mature and immature. Mature defenses can be seen in the general adult population and are regarded as healthy when used occasionally. Immature defenses are primitive and used by children and adolescents or by those with personality disorders.[1] Some common mechanisms are discussed as follows:[1]

- Mature defense mechanisms include
  - Altruism: Serving others to experience pleasure
  - Humor: Turning unacceptable thoughts or emotions into acceptable ones through the use of jokes or a lighthearted comment
  - Sublimation: Turning unacceptable thoughts or actions into acceptable ones, such as utilizing sports as an outlet for aggression
  - Suppression: Postponing attention to an impulse or conflict
- Immature defense mechanisms include
  - Denial: The refusal of a reality or fact that one does not want to admit to or deal with, such as denying the negative effects of smoking or other substance use
  - Regression: The return to an earlier stage of development when overwhelmed, such as resumption of thumb-sucking behaviors in a child who had previously outgrown the behavior
  - Projection: Attributing one's feelings or actions to others, such as a cheating spouse accusing the other of infidelity
  - Acting out: Using inappropriate behaviors to express emotions, such as slamming a door instead of verbalizing that one is angry
  - Displacement: Redirection of negative thoughts toward others who are not the cause of them, such as yelling at children after being angry with one's boss
  - Rationalization: Providing a different explanation once a reality has changed, such as stating one never liked his or her job after getting fired
  - Intellectualization: Overemphasis on thinking instead of experiencing
  - Dissociation: Disconnecting from the real world, which often occurs in individuals who are abused

DEFINITION OF MENTAL ILLNESS

Mental illnesses affect emotions, behaviors, and/or thoughts.[1] Patients may need to be educated about psychiatric illnesses as they relate to medical illnesses in order to facilitate understanding and decrease stigma. Just as patients need evaluation and treatment for asthma, hypertension, or diabetes, they also need evaluation and treatment for mood disorders, anxiety, or psychosis. Individuals are not "crazy" but are experiencing impairment in functioning due to a complicated interplay of biological, sociocultural, and psychological factors.

GRIEF

Grief is a common and natural reaction to death or loss. It is not a mental illness. Several theories of grieving exist, but perhaps the most widely known is the five stages of grief as described by Elisabeth Kübler-Ross. Initially meant to describe the process that one goes through when diagnosed with a terminal illness and facing death, the stages have since been applied to what others go through following a loss.[1] The stages include denial, anger, bargaining, depression, and acceptance.[1,7] Not everyone progresses through these stages, or in that order, but the stages comprise a framework for coping with loss, be it one's own terminal diagnosis, or the loss of a loved one. Individuals may spend either a brief time or a longer amount of time in a stage, and can return to a previous stage.

Denial is the first stage, which, as discussed earlier, is a defense mechanism to help cope with the shock of the event. It can be difficult to accept the news of one's own terminal illness, or the loss of a loved one.[7] Feeling numb and disconnected from the world is common.

Anger is the next stage during which individuals may use this emotion as a way to form a connection to something after experiencing the vastness of loss.[7] Anger toward faith or toward loved ones is common. Note that patients may displace their anger onto the clinician and that this should not be taken personally.[1]

Bargaining involves wondering "what if" or "if only" and can be accompanied by feelings of guilt.[7] Wanting to negotiate with clinicians, family, or God in return for a cure or a different outcome is common. Patients may need to be encouraged and to understand that regardless of their bargaining, they or the loved one will be taken care of to the best of the abilities of the treatment team.[1]

Depression in the context of grief is normal and expected. Symptoms include those that are seen in major depressive disorder such as sleep disturbance, hopelessness, or anhedonia.[1] If depression persists and criteria are met for major depressive disorder, this would be the more appropriate diagnosis.[1,7]

Acceptance does not imply that one is fine with the outcome, but rather indicates one is adjusting to the new reality without a loved one, or has accepted one's own terminal status.[1,7] Moving on with life may cause individuals to feel that they are betraying their deceased love one. Realizing that it is acceptable to develop a new routine or new relationship is part of this stage.[7]

Most agree that after approximately 6 months, the severity of the grief reaction following a loss begins to decline.[1,8] Complicated grief, or persistent bereavement, has been discussed in the literature. It is recognized that a portion of individuals continue to experience impairment from grief and may need to be evaluated for treatment from a depressive or traumatic perspective.[1]

MEDICATION COMPLIANCE AND RISKS

Many psychiatric illnesses are chronic, and remaining compliant with treatment is essential for optimal health and well-being, and to avoid hospitalizations or other complications. At times, compliance with various classes of psychiatric medications is difficult due to the adverse side effects they cause.[1] Patients need to be encouraged to discuss unwanted effects with the prescribing clinician so that attempts can be made to ameliorate them without compromising mental stability.

In addition to compliance, the risks of pharmacotherapy must also be included as part of informed consent. Some of the commonly used pharmacological classes are discussed as follows:

Antipsychotics

- Antipsychotic agents are utilized in the treatment of psychotic disorders, and some are used as mood stabilizers.

- A black-box warning exists for the use of antipsychotics in patients with dementia due to increased risk of mortality.[1,3]

- Atypical antipsychotics can impair insulin metabolism. Glucose, lipid, and weight monitoring should occur[1] in such cases.

- A risk of QTc prolongation exists with the use of antipsychotics.[1]

- Hyperprolactinemia can occur with typical (first-generation) antipsychotics and risperidone.[1]

- Quetiapine may cause cataracts; therefore, patients should be referred for a visual screening evaluation at the start of treatment and at 6-month intervals.[1]

- Clozapine carries a risk of agranulocytosis and monitoring of complete blood counts (CBCs) is required during treatment.[1]

- All antipsychotics have the potential to cause extrapyramidal side effects (EPS), but this risk is greater with first-generation (typical) antipsychotics.[1]

> **CLINICAL PEARL:** EPS include tardive dyskinesia, dystonic reaction, parkinsonism, or akathisia.

Benzodiazepines

- This class of medications is effective for anxiety but should be used in the short term or as needed due to risk of dependence.

- Side effects include
  - Drowsiness, dizziness, cognitive impairment, and anterograde amnesia[1]

- The use of benzodiazepine-like (nonbenzodiazepines, "Z-drugs") drugs for insomnia has resulted in rare reports of sleepwalking or performance of complex tasks without any recollection of the actions.[1]

> **CLINICAL PEARL:** Benzodiazepines should never be discontinued suddenly following regular use. Dependence can occur and withdrawal can be life-threatening.[1]

Bupropion

- Bupropion is an antidepressant in a class of its own.

- It is used as an alternative to treatment with a selective serotonin reuptake inhibitor (SSRI) or serotonin–norepinephrine reuptake inhibitor (SNRI) as it does not induce sexual dysfunction because it generally lacks these effects.[1]

- It is contraindicated in patients with a seizure disorder and/or eating disorders, as it lowers the seizure threshold.[1]

Mood Stabilizers

- These medications are utilized in the treatment of bipolar disorder
- Lithium side effects include the following:
  - Nausea, tremor, increased thirst and urination, and weight gain
  - Long-term effects can include hypothyroidism[1]
  - The therapeutic window is narrow, and toxicity can occur; drug levels need to be monitored[1]
  - Risk of congenital cardiac defects, including Ebstein anomaly in offspring if used during pregnancy
- Lamotrigine can cause Stevens–Johnson syndrome[1]
- Valproic acid can cause neural tube defects, mainly spina bifida, if used during pregnancy; valproate levels need to be monitored, as do CBCs and liver function studies (LFTs) [1]

SSRIs and SNRIs

- SSRIs and SNRIs are widely utilized in the treatment of depression and anxiety disorders
- Common side effects
  - Sexual dysfunction, gastrointestinal effects, headache, dizziness, or blurred vision[1]
  - SNRIs can also increase blood pressure[1]
    - SSRIs can have a paradoxical effect initially during which anxiety is worsened, and this can be mitigated by beginning at low doses and titrating up slowly.[1]

> **CLINICAL PEARL:** Educate patients not to stop these medications suddenly because a discontinuation syndrome can occur. This is not life-threatening, but can include influenza-like symptoms, insomnia, nausea, or paresthesias.[4]

Stimulants

- Stimulant medications are primarily used for attention deficit hyperactivity disorder (ADHD). Modafinil is used for narcolepsy. They have a high potential for abuse and diversion. Monitor for weight loss, hypertension, insomnia, and tics.[1]

Tricyclic Antidepressants (TCAs)

- TCAs are no longer first-line agents in the treatment of depression but are commonly utilized for pain.
- TCAs can be fatal in an overdose.[1]
- TCAs classically cause anticholinergic side effects.

> **CLINICAL PEARL:** Anticholinergic effects include blurred vision, urinary retention, dry mouth, and constipation.

PSYCHIATRIC MYTHS

There are some common misconceptions in psychiatry that you should be aware of and educate patients about:[2]

- Patients with psychiatric illnesses are not weak and can not just "snap out of it." Mental illnesses are caused by a variety of biological, psychological, and environmental factors. Although patients sometimes can work to improve coping skills, no one acquires a mental illness by being weak-minded or lazy.
- Treatment will not involve just taking pills or talking with someone. These modalities can be tailored to suit the patient and can include one, the other, or both.
- Individuals with mental illness are not crazy. Some psychiatric illnesses cause symptoms that seem strange or bizarre, but labeling individuals with derogatory terms ignores the evidence of the etiology of these illnesses and further perpetuates stigma. Many individuals with psychiatric illnesses are high functioning and do not behave bizarrely or inappropriately.
- Patients with mental illness are not more likely to be violent. A small percentage of violent acts are attributed to those with psychiatric disease. Many of these individuals are more prone to being victims of violent crime than perpetrators.

- Addiction is not caused by a lack of willpower. The etiology of substance use disorders is complex and involves multiple factors.

- Electroconvulsive therapy is not inhumane or barbaric. It is the most effective treatment for depression and can be lifesaving in patients who do not respond to first-line treatments.[2]

Substance Use Disorder Education

Individuals with mental illness are more likely to have comorbid substance use disorders.[1] This is referred to as *co-occurring disorders*. According to the 2016 Substance Abuse and Mental Health Services Administration (SAMHSA) report, 3.4% (8.2 million) of adults over the age of 18 had both a substance use disorder and a mental illness in the past year.[5]

Education about the risks and effects of substance use should occur with patients and families. They should also be made aware of the availability and efficacy of treatments, including psychotherapeutic and pharmacologic options, or both.[1] Medication-assisted therapy (MAT) exists for alcohol and opioid use disorders.[1] Several important patient education points are included in the text that follows, but please also refer to Chapter 2, Common Disease Entities in Psychiatry, for more detail on substance use disorders.

- Alcohol
  - Binge drinking is having five or more drinks for males, or four or more for females on the same occasion in 1 day[1]
  - "One drink" is
    - One 12-ounce beer
    - One 4- to 5-ounce glass of wine
    - 1.5 ounces (a "shot") of distilled liquor[1]
  - Significant medical complications occur with long-standing alcohol use disorder
- Caffeine
  - In high doses, caffeine can cause cardiac arrhythmias and should not be viewed as harmless
  - The most common symptom of caffeine withdrawal is headache[1]
- Cannabis
  - Patients can become addicted to cannabis

○ Motor impairment can occur while intoxicated, and patients should use caution while driving[1]

- Hallucinogens
  ○ The use of hallucinogens can result in a persistent perceptual disorder, with symptoms occurring when not intoxicated[1]
- Inhalants
  ○ A phenomenon, "sudden sniffing death," can occur[1]
- Opioids
  ○ Intravenous use increases the risk for cellulitis, hepatitis, HIV infection, and endocarditis[1]
  ○ Patients may inadvertently overdose in an attempt to get "high," and should be warned of this potentially life-threatening risk
- Stimulants
  ○ Cocaine and amphetamine substances can have significant side effects, including cardiac events and psychosis[1]
- Tobacco
  ○ Patients with schizophrenia have significantly high rates of nicotine use disorder; the reason for this is not completely understood; nicotine may decrease the concentration of some antipsychotic medications[1,6]
  ○ Patients need to be aware of the obvious negative effects of smoking or other tobacco use

WARNING SIGNS OF PSYCHIATRIC ILLNESS

Patients and families can be educated on potential signs of psychiatric illness, especially if there is a positive family history or other increased risk. The following symptoms may not always be indicative of a psychiatric disorder, but, if present, individuals can be encouraged to seek further evaluation.

- Apathy
- Appetite change
- Decline in functioning (at school, work, or activities) or personal care
- Difficulty concentrating

- Illogical or unusual thinking or behaviors
- Memory impairment
- Mood change
- Nervousness or anxiety
- Social withdrawal
- Weight change

REFERENCES

1. Sadock BJ, Sadock VA, Ruiz P. *Kaplan and Sadock's Synopsis of Psychiatry.* 11th ed. Philadelphia, PA: Wolters Kluwer; 2015.
2. U.S. Department of Health & Human Services. Mental health myths and facts. https://www.mentalhealth.gov/basics/mental-health-myths-facts
3. Steinberg M, Lyketsos CG. Atypical antipsychotic use in patients with dementia: managing safety concerns. *Am J Psychiatry.* September 2012;169(9):900–906. doi:10.1176/appi.ajp.2012.12030342
4. Warner CH, Bobo W, Warner C, et al. Antidepressant discontinuation syndrome. *Am Fam Physician.* 2006;74(3):449–456. https://www.aafp.org/afp/2006/0801/p449.html
5. Substance Abuse and Mental Health Services Administration. Key substance use and mental health indicators in the United States: results from the 2016 national survey on drug use and health. https://www.samhsa.gov/data/report/key-substance-use-and-mental-health-indicators-united-states-results-2016-national-survey
6. Khanna P, Clifton AV, Banks D, Tosh GE. Smoking cessation advice for people with serious mental illness. *Cochrane Database Syst Rev.* 2016;(1):CD009704. doi:10.1002/14651858.CD009704.pub2
7. Kessler D. The five stages of grief. https://grief.com/the-five-stages-of-grief
8. Moayedoddin B, Markowitz JC. Abnormal grief: should we consider a more patient-centered approach? *Am J Psychother.* 2015;69(4):361–378. doi:10.1176/appi.psychotherapy.2015.69.4.361

5

Urgent Management

Introduction

There are several situations or adverse medication effects that require urgent attention in the psychiatric setting. Patients may not be able to identify what circumstances necessitate an urgent or emergent need as easily as a medical condition such as chest pain or symptoms of a stroke. It is vital, therefore, that patients and those in their support system receive education on symptoms or signs to look out for. Prevention of tragedies such as suicide or homicide is possible with careful assessment of risk factors and proper intervention. Additionally, patients should be educated to be aware of potentially fatal pharmacological reactions. These syndromes, toxicities, or withdrawals need to be recognized and treated appropriately. Physician assistants will play a role in assessing and treating these urgent conditions in a variety of medical settings and specialties.

ACUTE DYSTONIA

Overview and Presentation

A dystonic reaction occurs as an extrapyramidal side effect (EPS) of antipsychotic treatment. It is reversible and can occur with either first- or second-generation antipsychotics, but is less common with the latter. It is more common in young males and with higher doses. It also more commonly occurs shortly after initiation of the drug and with a recent dosage increase. Other risks include a prior history of dystonia and a positive family history.[1]

Diagnostic Evaluation

The diagnosis is made clinically after the patient reports or is noticed to have a (typically) sudden onset of involuntary contraction of muscles, usually in the face, tongue, or neck. The eyes and trunk can be affected as well.[1]

Management

The dosage of the antipsychotic should be reduced and either benztropine (Cogentin) or diphenhydramine (Benadryl) is given intramuscularly.[1] A dystonic reaction is rarely lifethreatening but can be very distressing to patients.

AKATHISIA

Overview and Presentation

Akathisia can occur as an EPS of antipsychotic treatment. It is reversible and can occur with either first- or second-generation antipsychotics, but the risk is higher with the first-generation class.[1] As with a dystonic reaction, akathisia is more common at higher doses and with rapid dosage increases.

Diagnostic Evaluation

The diagnosis is made clinically after the patient reports agitation, restlessness, and muscular discomfort. Akathisia is unpleasant for the patient, and he or she may state that he or she feels the need to move. The patient may physically rock back-and-forth, pace, or shift his or her weight if standing. It can be common to attribute these symptoms to anxiety, and in response, increase the dose of the antipsychotic. Be mindful to carefully evaluate whether the patient is experiencing a need to physically move versus a mental anxiety.[1]

Management

The dosage of the antipsychotic should be reduced. Benzodiazepines, propranolol, benztropine (Cogentin), or diphenhydramine (Benadryl) are given.[1] Akathisia can be very distressing to patients and can even lead to SI. Making the diagnosis and initiating treatment are extremely important in avoiding tragedies.

DELIRIUM TREMENS

Overview and Presentation

The most severe and final stage of alcohol withdrawal is delirium tremens (DTs). Not all patients in alcohol withdrawal will progress to DTs, but it is a life-threatening medical emergency. Withdrawal seizures may precede the development of DTs, but not always.[1]

Diagnostic Evaluation

Symptoms include delirium, hypertension, tachycardia, diaphoresis, fever, and anxiety. Visual and tactile hallucinations are more typically experienced. Patients admitted to the hospital for other reasons may have an undetected alcohol use disorder and begin to have symptoms approximately 3 days after admission / after the last drink.[1]

Management

Prevention is essential. Patients in known withdrawal should be treated with benzodiazepines to avoid progression to DTs, but if the initial withdrawal went undetected, benzodiazepines are given at higher doses with supportive care and fluids.[1]

LITHIUM TOXICITY

Overview and Presentation

Patients prescribed lithium are at risk for toxicity. Compared to other mood stabilizers, lithium has a narrow therapeutic range of approximately 0.6 to 1.2 mmoL/L. Toxicity usually occurs at levels above 1.5 mmol/L. Lithium is renally excreted, and toxicity can occur with nonsteroidal anti-inflammatory drug (NSAID) or diuretic use (especially the thiazide class), or with dehydration from vomiting or other causes of fluid loss.[1]

Symptoms include nausea, vomiting, abdominal pain, diarrhea, tremor, ataxia, confusion, slurred speech, coma, seizures, hyperreflexia, or myoclonus.[1]

Diagnostic Evaluation

Lithium levels should be routinely monitored to assess compliance and evaluated for toxicity. In patients presenting with symptoms mentioned earlier, order a test of serum lithium level to asses for elevation.

Management

Lithium should be discontinued. Management might require treatment in the intensive care setting. Patients should receive aggressive hydration and renal dialysis may be necessary.[1]

MONOAMINE OXIDASE INHIBITOR (MAOI) HYPERTENSIVE CRISIS

Overview and Presentation

There is a risk of a hypertensive crisis in patients taking monoamine oxidase inhibitors (MAOIs) who ingest foods containing tyramine or who take sympathomimetic drugs. Symptoms include hypertension, headache, stiff neck, diaphoresis, tachycardia, visual changes, nausea, or vomiting.[1]

Diagnostic Evaluation

No diagnostic tests will confirm the diagnosis but they can be utilized to rule out other differential diagnoses.

Management

Management requires monitoring of vital signs and the use of benzodiazepines to avoid seizures and control blood pressure. Antipyretics and cooling blankets can be utilized if the patient has hyperthermia.[1]

NEUROLEPTIC MALIGNANT SYNDROME (NMS)

Overview and Presentation[1,4]

- Neuroleptic malignant syndrome (NMS) is a potentially fatal but uncommon side effect of neuroleptic (antipsychotic) medication. The exact pathophysiology is unknown but involves dopamine receptor antagonism. It can also occur with abrupt cessation of anti-Parkinson medications, such as levodopa.[1,2]

- Examples of neuroleptic medications include typical antipsychotics, such as haloperidol or chlorpromazine, and second-generation (atypical) antipsychotics, including olanzapine, risperidone, paliperidone, aripiprazole, ziprasidone, and quetiapine.

- Note that the antiemetic agents metoclopramide and promethazine are dopamine receptor antagonists and therefore may also cause NMS or EPS.

- NMS usually occurs within 10 days of starting the medication, but can also come about after years of therapy.

- NMS is characterized by the following symptoms:

  ○ Autonomic instability

    ▪ Tachycardia, tachypnea, diaphoresis, hypertension, or labile blood pressure

- ○ Hyperthermia
- ○ Muscular rigidity and bradyreflexia
- ○ Delirium or confusion[1,2]

Diagnostic Evaluation

The lab abnormalities are generally a result of rhabdomyolysis and include

- Complete blood count (CBC): Elevated white blood cells
- Creatine kinase (CK) or creatinine phosphokinase (CPK): Elevated
- Electrolyte abnormalities
- Blood urea nitrogen (BUN) and creatinine: Elevated
- Liver function tests: Elevated
- Urinalysis: Myoglobinuria

> **CLINICAL PEARL:** A helpful mnemonic (for the diagnosis of NMS) is **FEVER**:
>
> **F**ever
>
> **E**ncephalopathy (confusion)
>
> **V**ital sign abnormality
>
> **E**levated enzymes (CK, CPK)
>
> **R**igidity of muscles

Management

- Discontinuation of offending medication
- Supportive care: Hydration and cooling
- Consider benzodiazepines or dantrolene
- Future use of neuroleptics is not contraindicated

SEROTONIN SYNDROME (SEROTONIN TOXICITY)

Overview and Presentation

- Serotonin syndrome is a potentially fatal interaction between selective serotonin reuptake inhibitors (SSRIs) and other medications that increase serotonergic activity.

Symptoms include

- ○ Diarrhea

- ○ Restlessness

- ○ Autonomic instability that may resemble NMS

  - ▪ Tachycardia, tachypnea, diaphoresis, hypertension or labile blood pressure

- ○ Neuromuscular hyperreactivity

  - ▪ Tremor and hyperreflexia

- ○ Spontaneous muscle clonus

- ○ Hyperthermia

- ○ Delirium or coma in severe cases[1,3]

CLINICAL PEARL: A helpful mnemonic (for the diagnosis of serotonin syndrome) is **HARMED**:

Hyperthermia, Hyperreflexia

Autonomic instability, Agitation

Restlessness

Myoclonus

Encephalopathy (delirium/coma)

Diarrhea, Diaphoresis

Diagnostic Evaluation

Serotonin syndrome is diagnosed clinically. Labs may be ordered to rule out NMS as noted earlier. The increases in CK, liver functions, and white blood cell count will not be seen in serotonin syndrome.[1,3]

> **CLINICAL PEARL:** Serotonin syndrome can be distinguished from NMS in that it has a more rapid onset, the presence of restlessness or agitation, diarrhea, and neuromuscular hyperreactivity (as opposed to rigidity in NMS).[1,3]

Management

- Discontinuation of all serotoninergic agents
- Cyproheptadine (serotonin antagonist)
- Supportive care: Hydration[1,3]

SUICIDE RISK ASSESSMENT

Overview and Presentation

Unfortunately, suicide occurs even with the best of care; it is not possible to predict who will attempt or complete suicide. A thorough assessment of risk must be completed along with an appropriate history and diagnostic evaluation. Direct questions are appropriate and are not going to plant the idea of suicide for the patient.[1]

Some discussions of suicidal ideation (SI) distinguish passive from active thoughts. Passive SI implies that the patient wishes he or she was dead, but has no plans to act on these thoughts, but would welcome dying in sleep or as a result of an accident, for example. You should not consider passive SI any less dangerous or concerning than active SI, as the passivity may change without warning.

- In the United States, over 40,000 deaths per year, or approximately 100 per day, are attributed to suicide.[4]

- Suicide ranks as the 10th overall cause of death and the second cause of death in ages 15 to 24.[1]
- Most suicides occur in those ages 35 to 64 and the most common method is hanging.[1]
- Although women attempt suicide more frequently, men have higher rates of completed suicide probably due to the use of more lethal means.[1]
- The most common mental illness associated with suicide is depression, followed by schizophrenia.[1]

Diagnostic Evaluation

- **Risk factors**
  - Previous suicide attempt
  - History of abuse
  - Male gender
  - Social isolation
    - Single, widowed, divorced
  - Unemployed
  - Positive family history
  - Poor physical health/ comorbid medical conditions
  - Mental illness
    - Depression, schizophrenia, dementia, substance use[1]

Management

- Risk assessment, identification, and prevention
- Hospitalization (voluntarily or involuntarily) must be considered in the treatment plan
- Treatment of any underlying psychiatric comorbidity is essential
- A depressed patient with SI might be at increased risk for suicide after treatment is initiated; although it sounds counterintuitive, patients may experience an improvement in energy level, which then allows them to proceed with a suicide plan[1]; careful monitoring should occur

> **CLINICAL PEARL:** Self-mutilating behaviors such as cutting or burning may also be referred to as parasuicidal behavior. Individuals exhibiting this behavior do not typically wish to die, but may self-harm in an attempt to relieve tension or express anger at themselves or others.[1] These behaviors are common in borderline personality disorder.

TRICYCLIC ANTIDEPRESSANT (TCA) TOXICITY

Overview and Presentation

The use of tricyclic antidepressants (TCAs) has declined since the advent of the SSRIs in the latter half of the last century, but you may still find them used for depression or for chronic pain in adults, and for anxiety disorders in children. They work by inhibiting the reuptake of serotonin and norepinephrine. They exhibit anticholinergic action, and are also alpha blockers.

An overdose of TCAs can be life-threatening and will result mainly in anticholinergic effects. These may include cardiac conduction abnormalities, palpitations, chest pain, hypotension, respiratory depression, agitation, hallucinations, seizures, or central nervous system (CNS) stimulation or depression.[1]

Diagnostic Evaluation

Electrocardiogram monitoring should occur. Intravenous access should be obtained, and the airway should be protected.

Management

Activated charcoal could be considered if the patient is stable and it is within 2 hours of ingestion. Sodium bicarbonate might be indicated for dysrhythmias. Benzodiazepines can be given for seizures.[1]

USE OF RESTRAINTS

Overview and Presentation

- Restraints should be used as a last resort to provide a safe environment for patients and staff. If a patient is violent such that he or she poses a threat to himself or herself or others, restraints may be necessary if no other less restrictive alternatives are available.[1]

- Categories of restraints can include physical, chemical, or seclusion.

  ○ Physical restraint is the use of a device or intervention that limits movement. Physical restraints can be indicated in violent or nonviolent situations, such as to prevent patients who are confused or agitated from removing intravenous lines. Raising the bedrails, the use of hand mitts, vests (sometimes called "posey" vests, after the manufacturer), or belts around the extremities or waist can be considered physical restraints.

  ○ Chemical restraint is the use of a medication to restrict movement or behavior. Laws for chemical restraint use vary. Commonly used medication classes include antipsychotics and benzodiazepines.

  ○ Seclusion involves the involuntary placement of a violent patient in an isolated room.

- Patients can become violent for both medical and psychiatric reasons, and the use of restraints is not restricted to a psychiatric setting.

- You should follow the guidelines of the clinical site regarding policies of seclusion and/or restraint.[1]

VIOLENCE OR HOMICIDE

Overview and Presentation

Homicidal ideation does not occur exclusively in the context of mental illness. Several risk factors for the development of homicidal ideation are known, and are discussed as follows:

- Homicide is the second leading cause of death in those ages 15 to 25 in the general population.[1]

- It is a myth that patients with schizophrenia are more likely to commit homicide.[1]

- A past history of violence is the best predictor of future episodes.[4]

Diagnostic Evaluation

- Several risk factors for homicide include
  - Male gender
  - History of early aggressive behavior
  - Previous violent behavior
  - Victim of or exposure to violence
  - Substance intoxication or withdrawal
  - Antisocial traits
  - Poor academic performance
  - Association with gangs
  - Low socioeconomic status[5]

Management

- Assess risk

- Although not all homicides result from psychiatric illness, a threat made by a patient must be followed up and the potential for involuntary treatment considered. As discussed in the Introduction, in most states, grounds for involuntary commitment include potential danger to others.

- Most states have a duty to warn statute in which threats to a specific individual require intervention with law enforcement and notification of the intended victim.[1]

- Acutely psychotic or violent patients can be treated with antipsychotics and benzodiazepines.[1]

References

1. Sadock BJ, Sadock VA, Ruiz P. *Kaplan and Sadock's Synopsis of Psychiatry*. 11th ed. Philadelphia, PA: Wolters Kluwer; 2015.
2. Wijdicks E. Neuroleptic malignant syndrome. In: Aminoff MJ, ed. *UpToDate*. https://www.uptodate.com/contents/neuroleptic-malignant -syndrome. Updated May 31, 2019.
3. Boyer EW. Serotonin syndrome (serotonin toxicity). In: Traub SJ, ed. *UpToDate*. https://www.uptodate.com/contents/serotonin-syndrome -serotonin-toxicity. Updated March 12, 2018.
4. Centers for Disease Control and Prevention. Suicide: facts at a glance. https://www.cdc.gov/violenceprevention/pdf/suicide-datasheet-a.pdf. Published 2015.
5. Centers for Disease Control and Prevention. Youth violence: risk and protective factors. https://www.cdc.gov/violenceprevention/ youthviolence/riskprotectivefactors.html.

6

Common Procedures and Psychotherapies in Psychiatry

Introduction

There are a variety of procedures that may be utilized in the treatment of psychiatric illnesses. While pharmacotherapy is widely used, procedures such as electroconvulsive therapy are still used today. Others such as vagus nerve stimulation and transcranial magnetic stimulation continue to be researched and utilized more commonly.

In addition to procedures, there are several psychotherapy methods that are also recommended. Physician assistants should be aware of what options are commonly used by therapists and counselors, and the indications for use.

PROCEDURES

DEEP BRAIN STIMULATION

Deep brain stimulation (DBS) has been used for Parkinson's disease, dystonia, chronic pain, and tremors. It is also indicated for obsessive-compulsive disorder.[1] It is the most invasive of the neuromodulation treatments, requiring the surgical implantation of a device that sends electrical impulses to the brain through a generator in the chest wall. Risks during the surgical implantation include intracranial hemorrhage and anesthetic complications. Postoperative risks include hemorrhage, seizures, or infection.[1] Contraindications include structural brain lesions or significant injuries to the central nervous system. Current disadvantages include cost and logistics of care. Patients need to be monitored and potentially have device adjustments, which can be quite time-consuming.[1]

ELECTROCONVULSIVE THERAPY

Electroconvulsive therapy (ECT) is a noninvasive procedure that involves the application of an electrical current to the scalp to induce seizure activity in the neurons. It is most commonly used for treatment-resistant depression. Although it is known to be the most effective and rapid treatment for major depression, it is not recommended as first-line therapy.[1,2] Pharmacotherapy and psychotherapy are used initially. Other indications for ECT include mania, acute psychosis, intractable suicidal ideation, and catatonia.[1]

ECT was first used in the United States in 1940. Modern treatments are humane. Patients receive general anesthesia and muscle relaxants. The patient is to have nothing by mouth for at least 6 hours prior to the procedure. A bite block is used to prevent injury to the tongue or the teeth. Electrode placement is either bifrontotemporal or right unilateral. Seizures need to last at least 25 seconds to be effective. Treatments are usually given two to three times per week for a total of six to 12 treatments. They can be done on an inpatient or outpatient basis. To prevent relapse, maintenance ECT can be done as well.[1]

The patient's medication list should be reviewed. Benzodiazepines need to be withdrawn due to their anticonvulsant effect.[1] Lithium, clozapine, and bupropion should also be discontinued due to the potential prolongation of seizures or late-appearing seizures. In addition, theophylline should not be used because it increases the duration of the seizure.[1]

There are no absolute contraindications to ECT.[1,2] Caution should be used in patients with a space-occupying lesion due to increased risk for edema or brain herniation. Also, those with increased intracerebral pressure or those at risk for cerebral bleeding are at risk for exacerbating those conditions. Patients with a history of hypertension should be kept normotensive prior to treatment.

Common side effects include headache, myalgias, confusion, and short-term memory impairment, mostly as retrograde amnesia.[1,2] It is rare, but ECT can precipitate the development of a seizure disorder. Consent for ECT is needed just as with other medical procedures. The patient and family or others in the support system should be educated about the treatment's risks and benefits.[1]

Indications

- Depression (unipolar or bipolar)
- Mania
- Acute psychosis, including catatonia
- Patients with contraindications to pharmacotherapy treatment such as pregnancy, or medication comorbidities with drug–drug interactions[1]

PHOTOTHERAPY

Phototherapy, or light therapy, can be used in patients with a seasonal pattern of depression (seasonal affective disorder). Natural daylight, lamps, or other sources can be utilized for 1 to 2 hours per day to increase light exposure during the winter months. Phototherapy is well tolerated and may also have utility in sleep disorders and jet lag.[1]

Indication

- Major depressive disorder with a seasonal pattern (seasonal affective disorder)

TRANSCRANIAL MAGNETIC STIMULATION

Although ECT remains the gold standard for treatment-resistant depression, transcranial magnetic stimulation (TMS) is another noninvasive neuromodulation treatment that you may become aware of on your rotation. It may not be as readily available as ECT. In addition, it is not as effective as ECT but is less invasive.[2] The process of TMS indirectly induces small electric currents to the superficial cerebral cortex through the application of a magnetic field. TMS usually involves daily outpatient treatments totaling 10 to 30.

The treatments can last 15 to 45 minutes.[2] Unlike ECT, it does not require anesthesia, and the patient remains awake during the treatments. Risks include inducing a seizure. Complications include headache, light-headedness, and discomfort at the site of the magnet.[1,2] Contraindications include implanted or nonremovable metallic devices in or around the head[1]

Indication

- Second-line treatment for depression[1,2]

Vagus Nerve Stimulation

Vagus nerve stimulation (VNS) was initially utilized in the treatment of epilepsy. It later received approval for the adjunctive treatment of depression in adults.[1] VNS is not as effective as ECT, but has a role in patients who have not responded to less invasive treatments or ECT. The treatment involves direct stimulation of the left vagus nerve via a pulse generator, usually implanted in the left chest wall.[1] The chronic stimulation of the nerve fibers alters serotonergic activity in the brain. VNS is generally well tolerated. Side effects include altered voice, dyspnea, and neck pain. During the surgical implantation, perioperative risks are present, as are injuries to the vocal cords.[1]

Psychotherapies

Biofeedback

Biofeedback is a treatment by which one attains voluntary control of the autonomic nervous system. Instruments such as an electromyogram (EMG), EEG, or a thermistor provide feedback on physiological functions that the patient then attempts to gain control of and alter. This occurs through operant conditioning. Biofeedback can occur with or without relaxation techniques.[1,3]

Indications

- Anxiety
- Asthma

- Cardiac arrhythmias
- Hyper- or hypotension
- Incontinence
- Pain conditions
- Raynaud syndrome[1]

COGNITIVE BEHAVIORAL THERAPY

Cognitive behavioral therapy (CBT) is a common treatment that combines the techniques of cognitive therapy and behavior therapy.[1] It is indicated as monotherapy or in conjunction with pharmacotherapy for many psychiatric disorders. Cognitive theory posits that the way people think affects the way they feel. Behavioral therapy uses reinforcement to continue positive behaviors and discontinue negative ones. The goal of CBT is to recognize automatic, also known as *cognitive*, thoughts that are dysfunctional, and adjust the resulting behaviors to improve symptoms.[1] Examples include having a negative view of self in depression, a fear of danger in anxiety, a distorted body image in eating disorders, or the attribution of motor or sensory impairments in somatic disorders.[1] Patients may also experience faulty cognitive processes, including overgeneralizing, catastrophizing, or dichotomous thinking.[1]

Systematic desensitization, or exposure therapy, is a type of behavioral therapy for specific phobia in which relaxation techniques are performed in the presence of the anxious stimuli. The patient proceeds through steps that involve an increased exposure to the phobia, while learning how to relax with each exposure.[1] Exposure and response prevention (ERP) therapy is used in obsessive-compulsive disorder (OCD) to decrease or eliminate rituals performed in the context of obsessions.[1]

Relaxation training is another behavioral component that works to counteract the effects of anxiety. The goal is to reduce muscle tension, respiratory rate, cardiac rate, and blood pressure. Exercises that involve progressive muscle relaxation are common as well as yoga or Zen Buddhism.[1] Positive mental imagery is often incorporated into relaxation therapy.[1]

Indications

- Depression
- Panic disorder

- OCD
- Specific phobias (as primary treatment)
- Eating disorders
- Somatic symptom disorders[1]

DIALECTICAL BEHAVIOR THERAPY

Dialectical behavior therapy (DBT) draws from several other therapeutic techniques, including behavioral therapy. It is helpful for improving interpersonal skills and decreasing self-destructive behavior. Much evidence exists to support its use in borderline personality disorder. It is being utilized in other disorders as well.[1,4] The therapy can occur once a week, either individually or in a group setting. There is a group skills component, as well as individual therapy. Therapists can be available for telephone consultations as needed if patients find themselves in a crisis that could result in injurious behavior to themselves or others.[1]

Indications

- Borderline personality disorder
- Substance use disorders
- Eating disorders
- Schizophrenia
- Posttraumatic stress disorder[1]

GROUP THERAPY

Group therapy utilizes a variety of techniques and can also be employed within other therapies such as DBT. Goals of both the individuals and the group are its focus. Group therapy can provide a sense of belonging and support. Some groups allow appropriate confrontation by one's peers, which can assist the patient in enacting positive change. Insight can be improved upon when patients can listen to others with the same or similar problem. Peer-led, or self-help, groups such as Alcoholics Anonymous (AA) or Overeaters Anonymous are commonly utilized by patients as well.[1] Group therapies typically occur once weekly.

Indications

- Adjustment disorders
- Anxiety
- Personality disorders
- Phobias
- Psychosis
- Substance use disorders[1]

MINDFULNESS

Mindfulness is a meditative technique that has its roots in Buddhist philosophy. There is to be no analysis of or reaction to thoughts, just observation of one's thoughts and feelings. The focus is on a nonjudgmental state of mind during which one is "in the moment," or in the "here and now." Through meditation, patients can increase tolerance to anxiety or depressed emotions. Research has found that mindfulness is effective for a variety of conditions.[1,5]

Indications

- Anxiety
- Borderline personality disorder
- Chronic pain and other medical conditions
- Depression[1]

MOTIVATIONAL INTERVIEWING

Motivational interviewing is a method that helps individuals become internally motivated to change negative behavior(s). It is patient centered and can be used in the setting of substance use disorder treatment or other medical conditions. Strengths of the patient are discussed and readiness to change is explored. Through this method, patients become more aware of the consequences of changing behaviors, or not.[1,6,7]

Indications

- Substance use disorders
- Diabetes
- Heart disease
- Asthma
- Other mental and medical conditions[6,7]

PSYCHOANALYTIC THERAPY

Psychoanalysis is usually a lengthy therapy process by which repressed feelings or memories are brought to the surface into the patient's awareness, are expressed, and then resolved. It is valuable in discovering the unconscious motivators of behavior, but is less commonly used today.[1] Psychoanalysis can involve the common image of a patient on the couch with the therapist out of view. This therapy is insight oriented and therefore is not appropriate in acute psychosis or in a patient with impairments in daily functioning or relationships. Patients also need to be motivated to continue and work through this intensive therapy.

Indications

- Depression
- Anxiety
- Obsessions
- Clusters B and C personality disorders
- Sexual dysfunctions
- Conversion disorder

REFERENCES

1. Sadock BJ, Sadock VA, Ruiz P. *Kaplan and Sadock's Synopsis of Psychiatry.* 11th ed. Philadelphia, PA: Wolters Kluwer; 2015.
2. Lipsman N, Sankar T, Downar J, et al. Neuromodulation for treatment-refractory major depressive disorder. *Can Med Assoc J.* 2014;186(1):33–39. doi:10.1503/cmaj.121317

3. Schoenberg P, David A. Biofeedback for psychiatric disorders: a systematic review. *Appl Psychophysiol Biofeedback*. 2014;39(2):109–135. doi:10.1007/s10484-014-9246-9

4. Linehan M, Wilks C. The course and evolution of dialectical behavior therapy. *Am J Psychother*. 2015;69(2):97–110. doi:10.1176/appi.psychotherapy.2015.69.2.97

5. Rodrigues MF, Nardi AE, Levitan M. Mindfulness in mood and anxiety disorders: a review of the literature. *Trends Psychiatry Psychother*. 2017;39(3):207–215. doi:10.1590/2237-6089-2016-0051

6. Romano M, Peters L. Evaluating the mechanisms of change in motivational interviewing in the treatment of mental health problems: a review and meta-analysis. *Clin Psychol Rev*. July 2015;38:1–12. doi:10.1016/j.cpr.2015.02.008

7. Lindson-Hawley N, Thompson TP, Begh R. Motivational interviewing for smoking cessation. *Cochrane Database Syst Rev*. 2015;(3):CD006936. doi:10.1002/14651858.CD006936.pub3

7

Common Abbreviations in Psychiatry

AA: Alcoholics Anonymous
ADHD: attention deficit hyperactivity disorder
AIMS: Abnormal Involuntary Movement Scale
AMA: against medical advice
APA: American Psychiatric Association
BPD: borderline personality disorder
CBT: cognitive behavioral therapy
CNS: central nervous system
DBS: deep brain stimulation
DBT: dialectical behavioral therapy
DEA: Drug Enforcement Administration
DID: dissociative identity disorder
DSM: *Diagnostic and Statistical Manual of Mental Disorders*
ECT: electroconvulsive therapy
EEG: electroencephalogram
EPS: extrapyramidal side effects
GAD: generalized anxiety disorder
HI: homicidal ideation
HPI: history of present illness
ID: intellectual disability (formerly, MR—mental retardation)
IQ: intelligence quotient
LSD: lysergic acid diethylamide
MAOI: monoamine oxidase inhibitor
MAT: medication-assisted treatment
MDD: major depressive disorder
MHW: mental health worker
MI: motivational interviewing
MMSE: Mini-Mental Status Examination
MSE: mental status examination
NMS: neuroleptic malignant syndrome
NOS: not otherwise specified

OCD: obsessive-compulsive disorder
OT: occupational therapy/therapist
OTP: opioid treatment program
PANDAS: pediatric autoimmune neuropsychiatric disorders associated with streptococcal infections
PD: Parkinson's disease
PTSD: posttraumatic stress disorder
SAD: seasonal affective disorder
SAD: social anxiety disorder
SAMHSA: Substance Abuse and Mental Health Services Administration
SI: suicidal ideation
SNRI: serotonin–norepinephrine reuptake inhibitor
SSRI: selective serotonin reuptake inhibitor
SUD: substance use disorder
TAT: Thematic Apperception Test
TCA: tricyclic antidepressant
TD: tardive dyskinesia
TMS: transcranial magnetic stimulation
TR: therapeutic recreation
VNS: vagus nerve stimulation

Index